THE HIPPOCRATES DIET and HEALTH PROGRAM

Other Avery books by Ann Wigmore

BE YOUR OWN DOCTOR
THE HEALING POWER WITHIN
RECIPES FOR LONGER LIFE
THE SPROUTING BOOK
THE WHEATGRASS BOOK
WHY SUFFER?

THE HIPPOCRATES DIET and HEALTH PROGRAM

Ann Wigmore

WITH FOREWORD BY DENNIS WEAVER

AVERY
a member of Penguin Putnam Inc.

The medical and health procedures in this book are based on the training, personal experiences, and research of the author. Because each person and situation is unique, the editor and publisher urge the reader to check with a qualified health professional before using any procedure where there is any question as to its appropriateness.

The publisher does not advocate the use of any particular diet and exercise program, but believes the information presented in this book should be available to the public.

Because there is always some risk involved, the author and publisher are not responsible for any adverse effects or consequences resulting from the use of any of the suggestions, preparations, or procedures in this book. Please do not use the book if you are unwilling to assume the risk. Feel free to consult a physician or other qualified health professional. It is a sign of wisdom, not cowardice, to seek a second or third opinion.

Cover design by Martin Hochberg and Rudy Shur
Cover photo: Richard Tauber, San Francisco

In-house editor: Diana Puglisi
Typeset at TypeHouse of Pennington, Pennington, New Jersey

Library of Congress Cataloging in Publication Data

Wigmore, Ann, 1909–
The Hippocrates diet and health program.

Includes index.
1. Reducing diets. 2. Vegetarianism. 3. Food, Natural.
4. Reducing diets–Recipes. I. Title.
RM222.2.W454 1984 613.2'6 83-21455
ISBN 0–89529–223–8 (pbk.)

Printed in the United States of America

30 29 28 27 26 25 24 23

Contents

Dedication

This book is dedicated to you, in the hope that you will find greater health, peace, and happiness by its use.

Foreword

In the field of nutrition and health Ann Wigmore has made a special name for herself. Not one to follow others, she has pioneered her own path. First finding the answer to her personal health problems at age fifty using live foods and wheatgrass, she has a passion for her living foods diet. For twenty-five years she has shared her discovery with tens of thousands of people worldwide—including many who have been pronounced medically incurable. As a teacher and counselor, rather than a licensed physician, she makes no pretensions of recommending treatment or of making medical judgments. She is always quick in pointing out that given a chance the body will heal itself.

Vibrating with health and vitality, Ann Wigmore is constantly on the run. Reaching out to all that are open to hear what she has to say, she emphasizes through her program that anyone can live a healthier, happier and more fulfilling life. We are two people who listened, and who know she is right. We had been health-minded for over twenty years when we first met Ann, but colds, the flu, and other common health problems still plagued us. The idea that we could prevent even these minor imbalances was appealing, and we decided to give the Hippocrates Diet a try. We grew wheatgrass, sprouts, and greens, and made the juices and Rejuvelac. After four months of following the diet strictly, we felt fantastic. Our energy level was high and our thinking was clear. Since then we haven't suffered from even as much as a cold. And that was two years ago.

Now don't think that this is just another health food or diet book, because it's not. It represents a whole new way of living which can extend the length of your life—far beyond what has previously been thought possible. More importantly, it can improve your energy level and effectiveness no matter what your age.

We are pleased and honored to write an introduction to Ann's excellent new book. It has given us an opportunity to thank her publicly; not only for the health benefits that we and our friends enjoy, but for assisting many thousands of people around the world who have been relieved of the fear of pain and illness through her ideas. We plan to continue following the Hippocrates Diet for the simple reason that we want to feel like she does, perform like she performs, and look as good as she looks—at her age.

Dennis Weaver
Gerry Weaver
Malibu, California

1

An Apple A Day Or Have It Your Way

Beginning a new diet isn't easy, especially if it requires a lot of effort. Things like having to buy and eat exotic or dietetic foods, having to weigh everything before eating it, or having to serve yourself on smaller dishes to make starvation portions seem like a lot, are frustrating. And consider the reactions you get from your neighbors and relatives or family physicians who do not believe in the diet/health connection. Even so, probably the greatest hindrance to sticking with a new diet is a lack of results. Over the long run, most popular diets fail to improve health or foster permanent weight loss.

Why don't most diets work? Because they have been designed to make a buck, not to help the person who is serious about losing weight permanently and gaining health. Most of the popular diets are designed for people who have neither the desire nor the gumption to let go of the very foods that make them ill or overweight. These people resort to calorie counting, dangerous high-protein diets, costly and unnecessary supplements, or fad diets that encourage lavish culinary blowouts followed by days of eating nothing but fresh fruit in order to wash the bad food from the body.

The kind of food served at our "finest" restaurants or prepared by our prime time galloping gourmets is bad for us. The United States government has just completed two monumental studies linking poor food choice with the major killers—cancer and heart disease—that claim the lives of over one million Americans annually. In the first study, completed in 1977, *Dietary Goals For The*

U.S., hundreds of experts concluded that Americans eat too much sugar, salt, high-protein, and high-fat foods, and not enough fresh vegetables, fruits, and whole grains. The second report, *Diet, Nutrition and Cancer,* issued in 1982, goes beyond the first to single out meat, dairy, poultry, and other cholesterol-rich foods as contributors to the increased incidence of cancer, while fresh vegetables, sprouts, and greens reportedly help prevent cancer and other degenerative conditions.

What the experts are recommending is a wide, sweeping change in eating habits to include more Hippocrates diet staples—fresh vegetables, sprouts, greens, fruits, and whole grains. The problem is that we have gotten away from these wholesome, nourishing foods over the last one hundred years. Instead, the American diet has steadily degenerated. It has become more synthetic. The majority of foods sold at supermarkets today are heavily processed, even some of the fresh foods. Vegetables and fruits are canned, frozen, or irradiated. Grains are stripped of their fiber and twenty other nutrients, and then a handful of synthetic ingredients is added back to the "*fortified*" product. In addition, there has been a steady rise in the use of beef, pork, poultry, milk, cheese, eggs, and fish. As a result, over 40 percent of the calories in the American diet are fat, mostly saturated animal fat.

The high-fat, high-sugar diet is too rich for our bodies and we have a problem throwing off the excess calories, fats, protein, and minerals that often turn to fat or fatty deposits in our arteries. Our heavily processed foods also lack sufficient bulk to promote healthy bowel habits, so we turn to laxatives for help. Right next to the laxatives are the ever-popular antacid preparations used by millions of people to calm their upset, overacid stomachs. We do need dietary reform. In fact, we need a revolution in diet to correct the severe imbalances brought on by our modern food choices.

The Hippocrates Diet is simple and down-to-earth, yet it has taken experts years to recognize its value. Like our diet of one hundred years ago, it is rich in fresh vegetables, whole grains, fruits, seeds, and nuts. However, there is at least one important difference. Added to the already nutritious fruits and vegetables

are super-nutritious sprouts, baby greens, sea vegetables, chlorophyll-rich wheatgrass, protein-rich fermented foods, and fresh juices—as a group, perhaps the most nutritionally complete foods available. In addition, the Hippocrates Diet foods are eaten in their "live" or uncooked state: the vital nutrients they offer are unchanged. Cooking or otherwise processing foods destroys or leaches 100 percent of their enzymes, and to a lesser extent damages vitamins, minerals, and proteins, leaving some foods devoid of nutritional value except for calories. The differences between high- and low-quality proteins will be discussed in Chapter 5.

To be truly healthy and to ensure adequate protection from environmental hazards and pollution, it is important that you get an abundance of vital nutrients from live, uncooked foods and fresh juices. Of course, it is unwise to neglect fresh air, pure water, sunshine, exercise, and proper mental outlook as well. But a necessary and important first step is a healthy diet.

Fortunately, it's easy to begin the Hippocrates Diet. You don't take a blood test or a treadmill test; you don't need a heart exam or a physical. You don't need to check your blood pressure, or even lay a foot on a scale (although you may want to). On the contrary, all you need do is make the commitment to yourself that you will make your health improve through desire and a little effort. It's true, some effort is necessary; but starvation diets, expensive or dangerous chemical supplements, an hour of meditation, and a half hour of sunbathing per day are not necessary.

The Hippocrates Diet is for anyone who wants to improve his or her health, prevent illness, and live longer. Some people I meet, however, especially older persons, feel the diet is somewhat extreme compared to the foods they are used to eating. For them I have added transitional diet ideas which include a few non-Hippocrates Diet foods and some lightly cooked foods. Nevertheless, the Hippocrates Diet is, after many years of careful research, what I consider to be the healthiest diet in the world. And I encourage everyone to begin eating as large a percentage of the Hippocrates Diet staples as they can—fresh sprouts, greens, vegetables, juices, and fruits,—adding the transitional foods only for flavor.

The initial phase of the Hippocrates program is the cleansing phase, and it is essential in preparing your body for the building/maintenance phase, which follows. Newcomers to the diet will do well to begin by using more of the cleansing foods mentioned and less of the building foods.

Cleansing foods remove blockages to good health. In this process, your cells get recharged and your entire system gets a needed rest from digestion and elimination of heavy foods such as meat. In addition to the cleansing diet introduced here, there are a number of non-dietary techniques which will help speed the dumping of poisons from your body (see Chapter 4). Together, the cleansing foods and aids will prepare you for the building/maintenance phase, which aims to remedy dietary deficiencies, tone the metabolic and digestive systems, and keep you in vibrant health.

CLEANSING

I suggest that you stick to the cleansing regime for two to three weeks depending upon how you feel. If after a few days you feel terrible, the cleansing is probably going too quickly for you, and you should slow it down by adding some transitional foods back into your diet. If you feel no discomfort other than a little lightheadedness and mild fatigue, keep on the cleansing program for the full two or three weeks. During this time you will notice that on some days your energy level is super high and you feel like climbing a tree, while other days you do all you can to drag yourself to work. This fluctuation is a good indicator of the cycles of cleansing your body is passing through. As debris is released and removed from your system, your energy level surges, but as soon as your blood and organs of elimination become congested you feel tired again.

The recommendations for the cleansing diet, similar to the one I have served at the Hippocrates Institute over the years, are outlined below. Try to eat three meals each day, including breakfast of watermelon rind juice and watermelon red meat if available. If not, substitute apple or pear sauce or other fresh fruit in season, or take a green drink made from a variety of sprouts, greens, and vegetables.

Between meals drink Rejuvelac (a fermented wheatberry drink) or fresh juices or chew on some vegetable sticks. Try to include the following foods in your meals and snacks each day:

- 2–5 pieces of fresh fruit, preferably in season. Limit bananas and dried fruits (always eaten soaked, to renew their freshness) to 2 times per week.
- 2 large salads with a light seed cheese, vegetable, or avocado-based dressing.
- 6 or more cups of sprouts either in salad, in soup, or as juice.
- 2 or more green drinks made from 50% sprouts and greens, and 50% vegetables such as celery, cucumber, carrot, beets, and so on (see Recipes for ideas).
- 8–16 ounces of Rejuvelac (see page 110).
- 1–3 ounces of fresh wheatgrass juice.

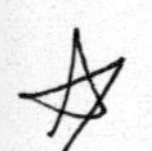

- 2 tablespoons of sea vegetables per day. To measure dried sea vegetables, cut them into small pieces and press them into the spoon. To use powdered vegetables, simply add 2 level tablespoons to the recipes you prepare during the course of the day. If your doctor advises you against the use of sea vegetables because of their iodine content and stimulating effect on the thyroid gland, do not use them.

Be sure to get plenty of rest, drink all the required fluids, and do some exercise each day, preferably walking and stretching. Also perform the non-dietary cleansing techniques discussed in Chapter 4 for insurance against uncomfortable reactions to the cleansing diet.

BUILDING/MAINTENANCE

Following the cleansing phase, I suggest the use of more high-calorie and protein-rich building foods. Combinations of sprouted grains, seeds and nuts, soaked dried fruits, avocados, and bananas are easily digested and nourishing foods. They are able to satisfy hunger as well as your body's calorie and protein needs. I also recommend the continued use of one to three glasses of mineral-rich green drinks made from vegetables, sprouts, and greens, and small amounts of wheatgrass juice. This might translate as sprouted wheat cereal with seed milk for breakfast; fresh juice and a large salad with a thick sauce and flat bread for lunch; and fresh juice or soup, sauerkraut, or cauliflower loaf, with salad and bread for dinner. Fresh fruits can be eaten between meals if you get hungry. Occasionally add desserts made from fruits, nuts, seeds, and sprouted grains to the menu for variety.

To get all the essential vitamins, minerals, enzymes, fibers, and calories, as well as amino acids for building/maintenance purposes, you should follow these basic guidelines for nutrition:

- 2–5 pieces of fresh fruit or soaked dried fruit daily.
- 2 large salads per day including a variety of salad vegetables and sprouts.
- 6 cups of fresh alfalfa, sunflower, buckwheat, mung, lentil or other sprouts either prepared in recipes or as juice each day.
- 3–8 ounces of seed cheese, seed sauce or seed yogurt made from sprouted or soaked seeds or nuts each day for added protein.
- At least 1 cup of one type of sprouted grain each day as bread or cereal, or in salads.
- 1–2 green drinks and 8–16 ounces of Rejuvelac each day. The green drinks may be used as soup. Carrot or other vegetable juices can be used occasionally in place of green juices. Drink fruit juice or cider less often.
- Sprinkle powdered dulse or kelp on food or add other sea vegetables to recipes 1–2 times a day (2 tablespoons in all per day), unless your doctor advises you against this.
- Drink 1-3 ounces of fresh wheatgrass juice each day.
- 3 or 4 times per week use avocado, sprouted or soaked nuts, soaked dried fruit and honey for added calories.

As long as each meal contains a combination of foods, eat until you're satisfied. If you get hungry between meals, drink Rejuvelac, vegetable, or green juice, or eat a snack of fresh fruit or vegetable sticks. If you eat three meals a day of the foods I suggest for building/maintenance, you should have no trouble maintaining your ideal weight. If you are attempting to lose weight, emphasize the lower-calorie vegetables, sprouts and juices, and eat fewer sweets and building foods. If you do not want to lose weight, eat more of the higher-calorie building foods made from sprouted grains, seeds, nuts, dried fruits, avocados, and bananas.

This basic diet will eliminate the need for costly and questionable supplements and calorie counting. Merely eat three meals per day until satisfied and add small snacks occasionally between meals. See the Appendix for a more complete breakdown of the nutrients obtained from an average day on the Hippocrates Diet. Beyond these basics, however, it is up to you to choose the variety, quantity, and the highest-quality foods available. I have listed my favorites in the Recipes. In addition, I have detailed the safest transitional foods to use on pages 53–55—those which are low in fat, adequate in protein, and rich in fiber. For example, a baked potato or a winter squash is a better choice than a hunk of cheese or sugary and oily baked goods. Ideally, even transitional foods should be limited to one or two moderate servings a day.

As you can see, the Hippocrates Diet is a departure from "Mom's cooking," but a necessary one for any person who wishes to improve his health and prevent further troubles. Dietary habits are thorny, but if you are willing to work at changing them, this book will guide you from sick to well, fat to fit, and sad to happy.

2

Let Food Be Your Medicine

The food you eat can be either the safest and most powerful form of medicine, or the slowest form of poison. Of course, food as medicine usually affects the body much more slowly than modern drugs. But in the end it can be safer and more thorough; it works by removing the cause of the illness, whereas most drugs merely relieve the outer symptoms.

"Let food be your medicine and medicine be your food," said Hippocrates of Cos (460?–377? B.C.), who clinically treated thousands of patients and kept detailed records of many of his cases. The records reveal a mixture of success and failure with the natural approach he preferred. In some cases he resorted to surgery and non-toxic herb drugs, but only in emergencies. In all cases, he attempted to understand the patient's life and psychology before prescribing any course of treatment.

Since the days of Ancient Greece, there have been hundreds of Western drugless healers who have had equal or better success than Hippocrates. And in the Orient, the famed Yellow Emperor and many other physicians employed natural therapies for thousands of years, dating back to at least 5000 years before the time of Christ.

Chemotherapy and surgical techniques, modern man's replacements for natural treatment, are still in their embryonic stages. It is a relatively new idea to use surgery to treat common complaints—and in some cases even to prevent problems. Having been used extensively for only the past fifty years, these techniques have had a variable success rate. Despite huge advances in the uses of surgery and chemotherapy over the past twenty-five years, life expectancy in the U.S. has increased less than four years on the average, while the death rate due to cancer, heart disease, and other degenerative conditions has risen sharply. Many synthetic drugs have been banned by the U.S. Food and Drug Administration (FDA) due to their numerous side effects. Thalidomide is merely the most notorious of dozens of these. On the other hand, penicillin, digitalis, and aspirin are examples of safe and effective drugs derived from natural sources. However, because even these drugs are more concentrated than the active ingredients found in foods or herbs, they have a faster action, are easier to abuse, and may produce side effects. One of the side effects that drugs are largely responsible for is psychological—our apathetic attitude towards self-responsibility in matters of personal health.

We no longer feel responsible for our illnesses. Microbes, germs, the weather, communism, or the wrath of an unfair God is blamed for the imbalance—and a miracle cure in the form of a pill is recommended as the cure. Rarely does the physician ask the patient to look at his entire lifestyle in order to find the source of stress, dietary or otherwise, that has created the problem.

We identify our bodies with simple man-made machines, that can only be fixed by an expert qualified mechanic. Like our broken cars, our broken bodies are brought to the garage (hospital) for repairs. But is the body a lifeless machine that breaks down with use? Do we really need an outsider's intervention to correct the common cold, a headache, or even more serious problems?

BODY AS SELF-HEALER

We all accept the simple fact that when we cut a finger or scrape a knee, our body begins repairs of the injury immediately. When the proper precautions are taken, there is no trace of any problem a few days later. Can we extend this seemingly simple, but in reality extremely complex, bodily response to other, more serious problems such as obesity, heart disease, diabetes, or cancer?

The fact that some people get cancer and fail to heal themselves by diet alone does not invalidate self-healing or natural therapy, but only the diet they are using. Obviously, the same diet that causes cancer cannot be expected to cure it, too. To prevent or reverse cancer with food, you would require a diet which contained many anti-cancer properties and high-quality nourishment. Yet, despite the thousands of case histories and mounting medical evidence to the contrary, many Americans have little faith in their ability to heal themselves when ill. You may be doubting it yourself as you read these words. But why does the human body, the very zenith of evolutionary development of Earth, fail to heal itself any more effectively than does the rabbit or duck? Can you name a single species of creature outside our own who, when hurt or ill, does not heal itself? We must remember that an animal's powerful instincts lead him to the cure. Civilization has all but snuffed out what little intuition or instinct we once had. We have become desensitized; lying helpless and hopeless, we submit our weakened bodies to specialists for care.

Your body can and will heal itself if given the proper nourishment, rest, and exercise. Every second you are alive, thousands of messages are being sent head to toe in an effort to maintain or restore balance in your body. If you are smoking a pack of cigarettes every day, your body may react by secreting excess mucus in the lungs to protect them (and you) from the vile smoke. Unfortunately, this emergency measure reduces vital lung capacity and slowly undermines the body's oxygen transport system, so that the smoker slowly dies by degrees.

According to a report by Drs. Lapage and Midler, published in *Cancer Research,* a high-protein diet can cause blood and cells to become too richly supplied with protein. When this occurs the lymphatic system attempts to remove the excess. However, if the burden becomes too great for the lymph to handle, protein "traps" (tumors) are created which are sealed off in order to protect the rest of the body from their contents. As Nobel prize winner Dr. Otto Warburg showed, when oxygen supply is decreased by as little as 30 percent, these trapped cells can become malignant cancer cells. Warburg found, that unlike normal healthy cells, malignant cancer cells don't require oxygen to reproduce. In a sense the cancerous cells consume waste, saving the body from poisoning by excess protein. But the body is also threatened by uncontrolled, terminal cancer.

For centuries, drugless healers have depended entirely on the body's ability to heal itself. By observing animals in nature—their often miraculous recoveries from accidents, poisoning or starvation—these practitioners have learned the efficacy of fasting and rest. Some animals use a partial fast and lots of exercise, while others prefer more rest and fresh grasses. In all cases, the only healing device the animals outwardly employ are food, rest and activity. Will not these same factors work to correct the many maladies endangering human health? Common sense, empirical evidence, and the personal histories of thousands of people say yes. Let's look at an example of drugless self healing.

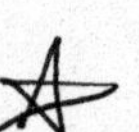

The Case of Eydie Mae Hunsberger

Eydie Mae Hunsberger and her husband Arn attended the Hippocrates Health Institute in 1973 because conventional cancer treatments were not helping Eydie, who had recently found out that she had malignant breast cancer. A surgeon she visited told her, "There is no known cure for cancer; we can't claim a cure. The best I can tell you is that you have an 80 percent chance to live one year, and a maximum life expectancy of five years." Eydie Mae chose to undergo a lumpectomy, which appeared to remove all of the cancerous tissue. But the cancer soon spread to other parts of her body. Depressed and confused, Eydie Mae and her husband Arn sought everywhere for help.

They met a woman named Wynn Davis whose son had died of cancer at age twenty-one. Her advice was to go to Boston immediately to visit the Hippocrates Health Institute, where Eydie might learn how to heal herself of the cancer. In a matter of days the Hunsbergers made all the arrangements and flew to Boston.

When I first greeted them they were both frightened and wondered if they were doing the right thing. Within two weeks, however, the fear and doubt passed and Eydie knew she would win the battle. Two years later, after sticking to the diet almost entirely, she recovered from her cancer. Her story is told in *How I Conquered Cancer Naturally*, by Eydie Mae Hunsberger and Chris Loeffler, Harvest House Publishers.

Eydie Mae's case history does not represent adequate scientific proof in itself. However, her experience and that of many others has given us observable evidence that the Hippocrates Diet can cleanse and strengthen the body when it is combined with proper rest and exercise. A stronger, cleaner system can better defend itself against the millions of germs, stresses, and potential carcinogens we are exposed to daily.

It would be fitting to end this chapter as we began it, with the words of Hippocrates: "Nature heals, the physician is only nature's assistant."

3

The Secret of Health

Nature heals and builds our bodies. But what is nature? How does it do the work? Surely not by some stroke of magic, or divine intervention. The secret of health lies in understanding the answers to these basic questions.

What is the great secret that has been eluding the investigations of scientists and lives of laypersons for centuries? Enzymes. You are alive only because thousands of enzymes make it possible. Every breath you take, thought you think, or sentence you read, is a result of thousands of complex enzyme systems and their functions operating simultaneously. Enzymes *are* "nature" or "metabolism," the body's labor force. They are the active construction and demolition teams that work twenty-four hours a day to maintain health and balance in your body.

Under even the best microscope, the miraculous enzyme appears to be little more than a protein substance. In reality protein is not the active agent of enzymes, but merely the material which stores the life energy of enzymes, just as a battery stores energy to light a flashlight. The activity factor (energy) of enzymes makes us living, feeling and thinking beings. Without enzymes we would be a worthless pile of lifeless chemical substances—vitamins, minerals, protein and water.

Unfortunately, life energy is not measurable by chemical or any other accepted scientific methods. Unmeasurable and unmanageable, enzymes and the life energy they represent are roughly charted territory on the map of science. Scientists have not yet been able to duplicate all their processes. For if they could, we might be able to create a piece of grass or raise ourselves from the dead.

We know life exists, that enzymes are the agent of life, and that all plant and animal life is a compilation of enzyme activity. But what do food and diet have to do with the failure of modern science to explain life, or for that matter, the activity factor of enzymes? Those scientists who fail to recognize and nurture the basis of life in humans, our hundreds of metabolic enzymes, also fail to see the value of the enzymes in foods and their relation to human nutrition. By and large, this has led to the devaluation of bodily enzyme functions, and the continued waste of our enzyme energy, especially in digestion.

Modern physiology texts claim that the body makes its own digestive enzymes to digest the food we eat. According to this theory, it matters little whether the food eaten is raw, with its enzymes intact, or cooked. But heat destroys all of the enzymes found in food. Of all the many thousands of species of creatures on Earth, only humans and their domesticated counterparts, house pets, attempt to live without food enzymes. And only these transgressors of nature's laws are so penalized with poor health. We cannot ascribe our present ills to vitamin, mineral, protein, fiber, or calorie deficiency because modern foods are well-fortified with these nutrients, and most people eat too much rather than not enough. We are, however, short on enzymes: metabolic enzymes, which run our bodies; digestive enzymes, which digest our foods; and food enzymes from raw food, which start digestion. Because good health depends on all of these enzymes doing an excellent job, we must ensure that we have and get enough of them.

Each of us is given a limited supply of bodily (metabolic) enzyme energy at birth. This supply, like the energy supply in your new car battery, has to last a lifetime. Unlike the car battery, there is no guarantee on how many years or months it will last. The faster you use up your enzyme supply, the shorter your life. The habit of cooking food and eating it processed with chemicals, and the use of alcohol, drugs, and stimulants draw out tremendous quantities of enzymes from our limited metabolic account. Frequent colds and fevers and exposure to extremes of temperature also deplete this account. With just scanty deposits—small quantities of enzymes from occasional salads and fruit—in time you create an imbalance and your body is ripe for illness. According to medical research compiled by the pioneering enzymologist Dr. Edward Howell, and published in his book *Enzyme Nutrition*, enzyme shortages are commonly seen in a number of chronic illnesses such as allergies, skin disorders, obesity, and heart disease, as well as in aging and certain types of cancer.

STORING ENZYMES AND ENERGY

The Hippocrates Diet stops unnecessary wastage of enzyme energy. At the same time each meal makes deposits into your enzyme account. Few withdrawals and large deposits are the key to becoming richly supplied with metabolic enzymes, the same ones that are responsible for building, cleansing, and healing your body. As I mentioned earlier, it is too vague to say "nature" heals, when it is enzymes that are doing the actual work. For example, enzymes break down excess fat to be eliminated in weight loss. An examination of the fat deposits of individuals weighing between three hundred and five hundred pounds reveals decreased levels of fat-splitting lipase enzymes. So if it is weight loss you are after, or reversal of any other form of deposit in the body such as calcium in arthritis, excess protein in tumors, or cholesterol in atherosclerosis, only enzymes do the work of breaking them up and eliminating them. Likewise, if you are in need of a few more pounds, stronger teeth or bones, sharper eyesight, or stronger muscles, only enzymes can help you. To include plenty of high-quality proteins, minerals, and vitamins in the diet will not do. Metabolic enzymes are required to build them into blood, bones, nerves, organs, and tissues.

As we age, our enzyme workers desert us: unless we do something to stop their one-way flow out of the body, our metabolic and digestive enzyme supplies diminish. This is what we call being over the hill—the entry point of a twilight zone of ill health. Of course, aging and death are inevitable, but when there is documented evidence that some inhabitants of the Hunza Valley in the Himalayan Mountains, and other peoples living in remote areas, live over one hundred and thirty years—in excellent health to the end—why do we settle for less? If the body is strong and healthy enough to reach beyond the one hundred mark, we will have much more mental and physical energy along the way.

It is not unusual to find wild animals living well beyond five hundred years in human equivalents. Does the lowly snake or primitive turtle possess some divine intelligence or supreme inheritance that we don't? Humans are the crowning glory of creation, far more complex than any other species, and yet, we settle for less vitality and length of life. Why?

GRAB FOR ALL THE ENZYMES YOU CAN

In following my line of reasoning, you may feel the urge to begin capturing the enzymes in your food right away. Food enzymes are the key to the Hippocrates Diet. Food enzymes, found only in uncooked foods, work to predigest food in the "food enzyme" stomach of a person or animal. That is, they help break down complex food molecules into simpler ones that are acted upon further by the stomach, pancreatic, and bile juices until eventually the food is absorbed in the small intestine. Nature's plan calls for food enzymes to help with digestion instead of forcing the body's own digestive enzymes to carry the whole load. If food enzymes do some of the work in the act of predigestion, the metabolic enzyme account can allot less activity to digestive enzymes, and have much more to give to the hundreds of enzyme systems that run the body.

All animals in nature are endowed with special anatomy for predigestion of the food they eat by food enzymes. A python can swallow an entire pig, but inside the snake few digestive enzymes are secreted until the final stages of digestion, which may take a week or more. During this period the dead animal's own enzymes, especially cathepsin, a protein-splitting enzyme, predigest its body and relieve the snake of the laborious task. In contrast, the average American male consumes 310 pigs if he lives to be 70, according to Dr. Saul Miller in *Food For Thought.* All of these are digested without the benefit of the pig's own enzymes.

Cows and sheep have a different mechanism for predigestion. As ruminants, both have four stomachs and chew their cud. The first three stomachs are for predigestion and the fourth is where the predigested foods are digested along with protozoa, tiny animals which the ruminant has in its first three stomachs to help predigest the grasses and other herbs eaten.

The chicken and other birds possess a food enzyme stomach called a crop. Seeds and grains eaten by the bird are mixed with saliva and sit in its crop for twelve or more hours. During this time the seeds begin to sprout. Sprouting starts predigestion of the proteins, starches and fats in the seeds and also neutralizes their enzyme inhibitors. These inhibitors, present in all, seeds, nuts, grains, and beans are nature's way of preventing their premature germination. (They are used up in the sprouting process as they are no longer needed by the growing plant.) In the bird's stomach, the germinated seeds or grains are then further broken down. For the bird, or any other animal living on seeds, beans, grains or nuts, predigestion and germination are essential; for when these foods are eaten raw, they contain enzyme inhibitors that block the absorption of their proteins.

The human food enzyme stomach is the cardiac (upper) portion of the stomach. It holds onto foods eaten for up to one hour, during which time a good deal of its carbohydrate (starch), fat, and protein content can be broken down. I say can be, because not all food is predigested. An enzyme-deficient meal of pizza, cola, a couple of twinkies, and a glass of pasteurized milk does not undergo significant predigestion, especially if the cola and milk are used like drain cleaner—to push large chunks of food down the tube. In contrast, a meal of salad greens and tomato, with avocado or lemon dressing, uncooked sprouted wheat bread, and raw fruit pie will undergo significant predigestion in the food enzyme stomach, relieving your own digestive organs and metabolic enzymes of the task.

On an enzyme-deficient diet, predigestion is minimal and the entire body adapts to allow for lavish digestive enzyme output. Most obvious are the changes in the digestive organs and glands which influence overall bodily functions. The pancreas, which secretes digestive juices into the small intestine, is an example. In modern man, the pancreas is two to four times heavier (in terms of percentage of body weight) than the pancreas of animals living on uncooked foods. The pancreas becomes larger on a cooked diet due to the body's increased need for digestive enzymes. But the pancreas does not manufacture enzymes any more than U.S. Steel makes steel. The latter brings in raw materials which it then refines and molds into steel products. Likewise, the pancreas gets its raw materials (enzymes) from the metabolic pool and transforms them into digestive enzymes. There is no proof that an enlarged pancreas is dangerous to health; however, wasting large quantities of metabolic enzymes for digestion is debilitating. For example, in extreme cases, where continuous vomiting is caused by gastro-intestinal obstruction, the individual will die in a week from loss of enzymes if the obstruction is not cleared.

The Pottenger cat experiment, which was published in several books and made into a film, has shown the superiority of the raw diet. Animals fed raw food produced offspring in successive generations. In the Pottenger study, which lasted nearly ten years, nine hundred cats were observed through four generations. The cats were split into two groups, the first getting only cooked meat and pasteurized milk while the others were fed raw meat and unpasteurized milk. The cats fed the cooked diet developed symptoms of all the major degenerative diseases found in humans. In each succeeding generation, the severity of illness increased. The third generation of cats that ate cooked foods was unable to produce offspring. Meanwhile, the cats fed the raw diet continued to produce litters of disease-free and healthy kittens for four generations, at which time the experiment ended. Further details on this study are available from the Price-Pottenger Nutrition Foundation, La Mesa, California.

The key to the success of the raw diet in maintaining health and healing is enzymes. Not only are the individual's internal metabolic enzymes preserved on a predominantly raw diet, but the need for digestive enzymes is also reduced. By giving the metabolic enzymes a "vacation" from their second job (digestion) they can be made more effective in their real job—repairing, cleansing, and building the body. But it is not enough to merely give the metabolic enzyme system a break. To be most effective it must also have assistance in removing the foreign matter and body wastes that have been stirred up by poor eating habits. In the spring when you clean your house you open all the windows and doors before sweeping the dust out. The Hippocrates Diet will stimulate the metabolism to give your body a spring cleaning; however, if the eliminative channels are not open and functioning well, it is like sweeping a pile of dust under the rug and thinking you have done your job. The waste may reenter the blood, bringing on a temporary return of past symptoms, leaving you feeling tired and uncomfortable. To avoid this inconvenience, we recommend a thorough body cleansing before you begin the diet.

4

Keeping Your Body Clean

Proper nutrition with enzymes intact is not enough to ensure good health and reversal of symptoms. A thorough body cleansing is just as important—and even necessary—before the vital nutrients in the Hippocrates Diet can be made available to your cells. By cleansing I mean the removal of metabolic wastes and excess accumulations of foreign matter such as protein, mucus, liquid, fat, calcium, and other minerals; metals like mercury, lead, cadmium, arsenic, aluminum; chemical residues from food additives, drugs, food sprays, and air pollution; radiation from X-rays, and so on.

Few, if any, people alive today can escape all of these hazards. In *Nutrition For A Better Life*, Nan Bronfen reports that "Contemporary American skeletons contain 500 times more lead than those of Peruvian Indians living 1800 years ago." Excesses of fat and cholesterol are commonly known to block arteries and blood circulation, while accumulations of certain metals can produce a wide range of allergic reactions in some individuals.

In this chapter you will learn how to help your body purge itself of residues which can block vibrant health. But before I give you the details of what you can do, it is helpful to have some background information.

Modern living has made it difficult for the eliminative organs—the colon, skin, kidneys, liver, and lungs—to function normally. Not only do they have to perform their ordinary cleansing functions, they must also contend with a diet composed of highly acid-producing animal foods and plant extracts, and the thousands of chemicals and additives in them. Our digestive system simply wasn't set up to perfectly separate the nutrition from the chemicals, and some potentially harmful residues may remain.

It is clear that Americans living an average lifestyle could benefit from a good cleaning out of the body at least every year. This probably sounds a bit strange, but would you let your home or car go unwashed or uncleaned for a year? What I am asking you to do is consider seriously the matter of internal cleanliness. Does the inside of your body ever become filthy? And if so, could it be more destructive to your health than external filth? Let's take a closer look.

Scientists estimate that each of us has over ten trillion body cells. While these cells are alive they are receiving a constant flow of nutrition which they metabolize into energy, carbon dioxide, water, and other waste products. The accumulation of wastes in the blood and organs can set up the conditions for toxemia, resulting in serious imbalances of the entire body.

The blood in our veins carries wastes to the organs of elimination. If these organs are functioning poorly because they are clogged with debris, they cannot remove all the waste from the blood. Unable to carry more toxins in solution, the blood forces the ten trillion body cells to accumulate waste to capacity. It is similar to what occurred in New York City during the garbage collectors' strike several years ago. The dumps were closed, not accepting any more garbage; and the sanitation collectors wouldn't pick up the trash. Buildings became overloaded with garbage, and then it flooded into the streets. Soon the city was filled with trash.

To clean up the mess it was necessary to open the dumps (organs) to allow the men and trucks to empty the trash they removed from the cans (cells). Before true health or reversal of symptoms can occur, waste products must be cleared from the cells, blood, and organs of the body. The sooner this is accomplished, the sooner the body will repair itself.

During the process of cleansing the colon, liver, lungs, kidneys, and skin, vital nutrients in the diet reach the cells and stimulate an increased metabolic rate. This speeds the elimination of waste products from the cells into the bloodstream, which in turn places a greater burden on the major eliminative organs.

My experience at the Institute has shown that some people's eliminative organs are not functioning well enough to handle an increase in waste without outside help. In fact, unless you aid the eliminative organs in their cleansing function, you may not feel well, and your body cells may not be able to fully utilize the vital nutrients furnished by the Hippocrates Diet. To avoid such uncomfortable, though ultimately positive reactions, it is important to assist your major eliminative organs during the first few weeks of the diet, especially the large intestine (or colon). Beginning with the colon, let us take a brief look at why this is so.

CLEANSING THE COLON

The colon is the body's main avenue for physical elimination of waste. The modern sedentary lifestyle, characterized by a diet high in animal fats, proteins, and artificial and refined foods, has made the colon resemble a sewer system. Like a cesspool, it may breed millions of harmful bacteria and emit foul and embarrassing gasses. Adding a few tablespoons of bran and a bottle or two of prune juice to the ordinary diet is not enough to bring an unclean or diseased colon back to healthy functioning. What is needed is a systematic program of diet, exercise and cleansing techniques specifically aimed at purging and strengthening the colon. Let's take a look at why.

All of us have used antibiotics, either directly to combat an infection, or indirectly in our food supply. Indirectly, we consume the tons of antibiotics that are fed to animals each year as an inexpensive way to fatten them for market. Inside the body, these antibodies destroy the sensitive and friendly lactobacillus family of bacteria, clearing the way for their replacement by putrefying and disease-producing bacteria and waste. Toxins like nitrosamines, ptomaines, and others can be reabsorbed through the colon into the bloodstream.

Common staples of the American diet, such as white bread, cakes, cookies, meat, milk, doughnuts, spaghetti, and overcooked vegetables, are fiber-poor foods that make it harder for the colon to do its job. The high pressures needed to move the remnants of a fiber-deficient meal through the colon remind me of the effort required to squeeze the last drops of toothpaste from the tube. Eventually, the lack of healthy bacteria in the colon, combined with the constant stress from fiber deficiency, can cause bubble-like blowouts, known as diverticula, in the colon wall. Medical research indicates that nearly all Americans over age thirty-five have diverticula. And while they are considered normal by some doctors, they can become infected and create the precondition for colon-rectal cancer.

Because of these dietary hazards, a little bran is not enough. The colon needs plenty of fiber-rich raw fruits, vegetables, sprouts, greens, seeds, nuts, and germinated grains. The Hippocrates Diet uses certain fermented foods such as saltless sauerkraut and pickles, seed and nut ferments, and Rejuvelac, that feed the friendly lactobacillius bacteria in the colon and help to cleanse it of harmful and putrefactive types. Some people who begin adding these—and the foods mentioned above—to their diet, experience temporary digestive upset. This is usually due to the stirring up of toxins in the blood and organs, along with the injection of food enzymes to the intestinal tract. The battle which ensues between the healthy and harmful bacteria doesn't last long, though, and can be eliminated altogether with the use of daily enemas for a week or two.

Enemas

The topic of enemas is not a popular one. If there was another way to accomplish the same end, I would be the first to recommend it; however, there is little doubt that a full enema is the quickest and easiest way to unblock a congested colon. And this may be necessary, especially during the first two weeks or so of the Hippocrates Diet, when sticky debris is sent to the colon from all parts of the body for elimination.

Enemas and colonics help to stimulate peristaltic activity of the muscles that contract the colon wall, thereby loosening deposits, which may be seen later (in the bowel) as hardened black material and ropes or lumps of mucus. A colonic is a continuous enema administered by a professional health care provider. One or more colonics per week can be used during the first month with occasional use when necessary afterwards. The use of wheatgrass juice in the enema water or as a wheatgrass implant, has an even more powerful action on the colon muscles than plain water. The high magnesium content of the wheatgrass juice also purges the liver of its toxic wastes. An implant using wheatgrass juice is in my opinion safer than the coffee enemas that are used by many health clinics, because wheatgrass does not introduce unwanted caffeine into the body.

All this talk about enemas and implants may have you cringing in your chair. If you have a psychological barrier against them, it will help to remind yourself that the removal of toxic matter from the colon is essential in healing. If you can then bring yourself to use them you will find relief and a sense of internal cleanliness that is refreshing. Of course, if you have one or two healthy bowel movements a day without them, enemas and implants may not be necessary at all. But they are good for most people, and in a short time they will help you to regain normal muscle tone and strength of the colon.

It is best to use the enema, followed by a wheatgrass implant, early in the morning. If this is not possible, or if repetition is desired, early afternoon or evening are also good times.

How to Take an Enema

A full enema can be self-administered using a sterilized colon tube attached to an enema bag filled with water (usually one to two quarts). Although 18″ or 20″ colon tubes are available, never force the tube in farther than it will comfortably go. While lying on your back on a slanted board or with a pillow under your buttocks, allow the water to slowly enter the colon. Do not force in more water than feels comfortable. Try letting the water in while you exhale, stopping the flow when inhaling.

Let in as much water as you can comfortably retain and gently massage your abdomen from left to right for two to three minutes. Then roll over onto your right side for a couple of minutes and repeat. This will allow the water to move along the entire length of the colon. Let the water come out when you feel the urge. Never force it to stay in. You can always repeat the process. If gas seems to be a problem, try removing the air from the enema bag and colon tube before inserting it in the rectum.

Rejuvelac can be used in the enema to help loosen the stool and restore the intestinal flora, as can wheatgrass juice.

Wheatgrass Implants

A wheatgrass implant is effective either as an immediate purge or as a retention enema. The juice may be retained for up to an hour before being expelled. Usually one implant per day is sufficient, but in extreme cases, they can be used every hour or two until pain dissipates. The implants work to purge the colon and liver and to nourish the body via absorption in the colon. Just inside the rectum (where the juice is inserted) lies the hemorrhoidal vein, which enters into the portal circulation. The portal vein receives liquids, minerals, nutrients, and sometimes toxins from the colon and transports all of these directly to the liver where they are either used or eliminated from the body. Since a portion of the wheatgrass juice is thus absorbed into the system, it works on the entire length of the colon and small intestine (and body), and not only on the lower bowel.

Many students at the Institute have found wheatgrass implants to be more effective than enemas in purging the colon, with half the fuss.

How to Take a Wheatgrass Implant

To use wheatgrass juice implants as a purge, simply fill a sterilized infant enema syringe with one to two ounces of fresh juice and insert it into the rectum. A couple of minutes later, the bowels will move hurriedly. Try another one to two ounce implant and also let it out if it wants to come. The second attempt will probably carry more fecal matter with it. A third implant, of two to four ounces will usually be retained with ease. Hold it in until you feel the urge to eliminate, generally about twenty minutes later. There is no danger of reabsorbing toxins if you have purged the colon first with other implants or enemas. You may even be surprised to find that all the juice has been totally absorbed inside you.

To perform the implant after you have cleansed the colon, simply lean to one side while on the toilet seat and use an infant enema syringe to squeeze the juice into the rectum. Syringes are available at most drug stores and are shaped like a small bulb with a removable hard plastic tip. Make sure that all the equipment you use is sterile. Three or four ounces of juice can be comfortably retained in the colon.

Try to hold the juice fifteen minutes to an hour before expelling it. If you forget about it, don't worry. I have used implants before bed at night, retaining them during sleep. Wheatgrass implants can be used during a health crisis such as the common cold or pains, every two hours or whenever you feel one is necessary. They can also be used effectively during days of fasting on raw juices.

Exercises For the Colon

One of the most important colon exercises is not actually an exercise at all, but the natural method of defecation for millions of people—squatting. Modern toilets and our normal sitting position close a portion of the colon, making complete elimination difficult. Squatting or placing your feet on an elevated platform opens the colon, allowing better and more complete evacuation. It strengthens the abdominal muscles, too, protecting you against hernias and hemorrhoids.

Some toilets in Europe are built into the ground with handles for the individual to hold onto while squatting over them. In your home you can put your feet up on the toilet bowl itself and squat over the bowl. An alternative method is to purchase or build a 10″ stand, place it in front of the toilet, and rest your feet on it while eliminating.

Another excellent exercise for the colon is the abdominal lift. To do this, bend over slightly, placing your hands just above your knees. Now, blow all the air out of your lungs, forcibly, and hold it out. A natural vacuum will be created, and with it, suck up your abdomen, pulling the stomach muscles in. If you have ever had to suck in your stomach to get on a pair of tight pants, you will know what the "in" part of the exercise is like. Relax without inhaling, to push the stomach out. While holding your breath, try to make your stomach as large and round as possible. This movement should be performed ten times. Then stand and breathe slowly and deeply. When you are ready, do another set of ten, and repeat until you have performed three or four sets of ten in all.

It is best to practice the abdominal lift first thing upon arising or between meals—never on a full stomach. The exercise is especially good if you have lost tone. It will gently massage and tone all of the internal digestive and eliminative organs.

The small intestine is where vital minerals, liquids, and, unfortunately, unwanted toxins are absorbed. The colon is the final stage of digestion before waste is eliminated. The nutrients (and toxins) are sent to the liver where they are reorganized, stored, and either sent out into the blood or out from the body. Toxins absorbed along with the nutrients are neutralized by the liver and transported to the kidneys for excretion. Eventually, all the blood and food passes through the liver for cleansing and renewal. I believe that in many senses, the liver is the master controller of all the bodily functions, depending upon the other glands, organs of elimination, and circulation to carry out its vital roles.

CLEANSING THE LIVER

Since the liver is the major organ of detoxification, it determines the health of the other organs and the blood. The liver is a processing plant and storage place for metabolic wastes and pollutants, as well as many nutrients. The foods of the modern diet, especially meats, fried foods, refined oils, and foods with chemical additives weaken the liver. Alcohol, tobacco and environmental pollutants add extra duties to the 260 known functions of the liver.

Bile, which is stored in the gall bladder, acts as a carrier for all liver wastes, including excessive cholesterol. It is also necessary for proper digestion and assimilation of fats. A fiber-poor, mineral-deficient, and refined diet tends to produce solid particles from bile components. We call these gallstones. But before stones are formed, weakening of the liver, due to partially obstructed bile flow, may occur. Symptoms such as skin problems, poor eyesight, hair loss and hemorrhoids may be present as the liver becomes stagnant and congested.

To regain health and energy, the liver and gall bladder must be cleansed and kept free-flowing. The highly touted oil-based liver flush is an extreme method which may leave one feeling very sick. Instead, at the Hippocrates Institute we recommend a somewhat slower and safer course of action, the steady and consistent use of moderate quantities of the juices listed below.

- Wheatgrass juice, the chlorophyll extract of 7-day-old wheat plants, contains an abundance of magnesium, enzymes, chlorophyll proteins, and a full range of vitamins and minerals (see page 93).
- Green drinks, rich in vitamins, minerals, and chlorophyll protein, are made from sprouts, greens, some vegetables, and if desired, a little sauerkraut juice.
- Lemon juice is a well-known and commonly used cleansing agent that contains citric and other acids that have an antiseptic action.
- Carrot juice, high in pro-Vitamin A, has a beneficial effect on the liver and stimulates the flow of bile.
- Beet juice, high in vitamins A, C, B_2, B_6, and folic acid, and minerals such as sodium, iron, calcium, phosphorous, and potassium, has a stimulating and fortifying effect on the gall bladder, liver, and kidneys. Take small quantities and sip slowly to avoid extreme reactions to its use.
- Apple juice, or fresh cider, is high in malic acid, pectins, and enzymes that act as a bile solvent and liver stimulant.

Juices are best taken either first thing in the morning or thirty minutes before eating, as a cocktail. Wheatgrass and beet juice are the two most powerful cleansers of the five listed and should be used in small quantities, sipped slowly. Green drinks are very important as they contain portions of all the other juices.

Newcomers to fresh juices should move into them slowly or dilute them with water fifty-fifty if they experience loosened bowel movements or mild feelings of nausea. Although such reactions are rare, temporarily cut back on the juices if they occur.

CLEANSING THE LUNGS

Without food we can live for months and without liquids we can survive for days, but breath is life. Without breathing, we can live only a few minutes. Perhaps this is the reason that almost all ancient cosmologies and religions made so many references to the breath. Breathing is our link with the atmosphere, the ocean, and the trees and plants whose leaves convert human carbon dioxide waste into a fresh supply of oxygen. When our lungs are congested with mucus and burdened by excessive carbon waste products, our vital lung capacity is reduced and we no longer have sufficient amounts of oxygen to burn up bodily wastes.

With each breath there is an exchange of gasses in the lungs. The venous blood is cleansed of its carbon dioxide and other waste products. A fresh supply of oxygenated air is absorbed into the arterial blood and delivered to all the cells of the body. Each day, thousands of quarts of air are purified by our lungs.

One effect of dairy products, baked and refined flour products, smoking and air pollution, is to create excessive accumulations of mucus in the sinuses and bronchial tubes. The build-up of mucus inhibits the cleansing function of the lungs and puts strain on the other organs of elimination—colon, skin, kidneys, and liver—to pick up the slack. If you have a mucus problem, it is especially important to avoid mucus-forming foods.

Anti-mucus foods and simple breathing exercises are the recommended cleansing regime for the lungs. Moderate use of foods such as raw green onions, garlic, horseradish and fresh ginger will help to cut down mucus. Other less pungent vegetables such as bok choy, daikon radish, lettuce, celery, cucumber, and watercress also cleanse the lungs. Wheatgrass juice is yet another excellent cleansing food for the lungs.

Similar in chemical makeup to red blood cells (see page 90), chlorophyll has been known to increase the red blood cell count in both humans and animals, enabling the blood to carry more oxygen and remove more waste.

The processes by which chlorophyll increases red blood cell count are as yet unknown. Despite some research results showing the ability of chlorophyll to do this, there is no definitive explanation.

Dr. Yoshihide Hagiwara, a Japanese scientist and health educator, has an interesting theory. He reasons that since chlorophyll is soluble in fat particles, and since fat particles are absorbed directly into the blood via the lymphatic system, that chlorophyll can also be absorbed in this way. It is his opinion that inside the body a conversion takes place enabling it to replace the magnesium ion in chlorophyll with an iron particle, making new blood. Only time and more research into the question will resolve the mystery of why chlorophyll works as it does. I will have more to say about wheatgrass, chlorophyll, and the blood in Chapter 8.

After beginning the Hippocrates Diet, you may notice an offensive odor on your breath. Since it comes from the bloodstream, and indicates detoxification via the lungs, superficial remedies such as toothpaste and mouthwash will not remove it for long. Be assured, however, that when the blood is finally relieved of its waste, your breath will be sweeter than ever.

Breathing Exercises

The body's supply of oxygen is largely responsible for the oxidation or burning up of toxins. Most adults use only one-quarter of their lung capacity when breathing normally. However, during breathing exercises, at least three-quarters of this capacity is put to use, adding a tremendous amount of oxygen to the blood. In fact, if you are new to deep breathing, the release of added oxygen into the blood could leave you feeling lightheaded.

Deep breathing should begin in the stomach, pushing the diaphragm down and out. Make sure you are sitting comfortably, with the spine erect and the entire body relaxed. Now let the inhaled air fill the middle and upper regions of the lungs. You will notice the abdomen automatically contracting and the shoulders going back as you fill the upper chest. Then, without holding your breath, release the air slowly, in reverse order, contracting the chest first, then the abdomen. If you become lightheaded and dizzy, stop. Otherwise, repeat this full breath fifteen times. Rest for five minutes and repeat.

It may be helpful to imagine your breath as a wave which rolls slowly into the abdomen, filling it up to the chest; then even more slowly rolling back out to sea, as the chest and abdomen are emptied. Most importantly, use some of the time you set aside for this breathing exercise to rest and recede from the thoughts and worries of the day. Try to be happy knowing that you are doing something good for yourself, and therefore benefiting your family and friends too.

CLEANSING THE KIDNEYS

Every day, four thousand quarts of blood flow through your kidneys, where it is cleansed of metabolic waste. Urea, uric acid, excess water and other metabolic waste products are eliminated and the acid-alkaline balance of the blood is maintained by the kidneys. Without their vital cleansing assistance, you would die of autointoxication in a few hours. Body temperature is also regulated by the kidneys. Considered "the seat of life" by Oriental doctors, the kidneys are believed by many people to be closely linked with reproductive functions and willpower. They are also responsible for eliminating drugs, pollutants, and bacterial waste from the body.

The kidneys are perhaps the most stressed of all organs in modern people. With several thousand additives and drugs finding their way into our food and water, the kidneys have an extra full-time job. Inside each kidney, millions of vitally important little filters called nephrons are damaged by the toxins. Unfortunately, many people don't experience symptoms of kidney damage until 90 percent of the function is gone, and then the damage is irreversible.

The first step in healing the kidneys is to avoid all refined, processed foods, salt, meat, coffee, tea, alcohol, tobacco, and tap water. The regimen we recommend for strengthening and cleansing the kidneys is safe and effective. The active elements in this procedure are listed below.

- Green drinks (see section on the liver).
- Wheatgrass juice acts as a diuretic and stimulant for increased kidney filtration of waste. Its chlorophyll content helps rebuild the blood and relieves the kidneys of their burden.

- Watermelon juice is an effective diuretic that is used every morning at the Institute for breakfast. If possible, obtain organically-grown melons; juice the rind, seeds and all. Watermelon juice helps to reverse fluid retention.
- Lemon juice is mildly diuretic and antiseptic. It may be put on salads or in water.
- Beet juice tones the kidneys. Try juicing the beet greens also. Sip small quantities or add to other juices.
- Sea vegetables provide vital minerals necessary for detoxification and stimulation of kidney functions. Up to 2 tablespoons of arame, dulse, wakame, nori, hiziki, kombu, or kelp can be used each day. It is better to use a variety of sea vegetables rather than just one type. Either whole sea vegetables or powdered forms may be used. Soaking unpowdered sea vegetables for 10–20 minutes before eating will lower their salt content.

CLEANSING THE SKIN

Your skin is a living organ. In fact, it is the largest eliminative organ of the body. To close the pores of your skin for even a few minutes, as depicted in the James Bond thriller, *Goldfinger*, could cause death. Nearly five pounds of waste material (mostly water) leaves our skin each twenty-four hour period, compared with about two pounds each via the kidneys, lungs, and colon. Clogged or inactive skin places a tremendous burden on the other organs of elimination. Conversely, healthy skin has the ability to work overtime, acting as a third kidney, as in the case of high fever.

During the process of bodily cleansing, healthy skin takes an active role. If eruptions, odors, unusual colors, and blemishes appear, this is a sign that the blood and lymph are being purged of waste. Once they are cleansed, these conditions will disappear.

Every twenty-seven days we have an entirely new skin surface. Unlike the snake's, our skin comes off cell by cell and is not usually noticed. Overly dry skin probably means that it is inactive as an eliminative organ. To open pores up, brushing the skin in the morning before showering and vigorous use of a loofah sponge in the shower are excellent. Look for a soft vegetable-bristle brush at a health food store. Often these brushes come with a long handle for scrubbing the back. This brush should first be used dry, from head to toe. Follow the dry brushing with a shower and rub the skin again, this time with a loofah, to remove the dead cells loosened by the dry brush.

Avoid the use of ordinary animal fat or detergent soaps. Instead, use a small amount of liquid castile soap (available at health food stores). Castile bar soap or kosher soap is also fine, but the liquid soaps rinse off more easily and more completely. Heavy soaping removes valuable skin oils and destroys the skin's beneficial acid mantle. To restore the latter, the skin must borrow extra Vitamin C from the blood and organs. A natural shampoo and conditioner are also recommended for keeping the hair clean. For a special treatment, rub two ounces of fresh wheatgrass juice into your scalp, leave it on until it drys, then rinse it out. The juice will stimulate circulation in the scalp and remove excess sebum.

Alternating warm and cold water flow just before finishing your shower will stimulate the pores in the skin to activity. If you are daring—and accustomed to the warm and cool treatments—try making the warm hotter and the cool colder. Be careful, however, that you do not leave the cold water on long enough to catch a chill internally. You should leave the shower feeling vitalized and warm all over.

Another excellent skin care technique is massage. Try to convince a friend, or your spouse, to exchange a weekly massage with you. If you are not sure how to proceed, borrow a massage book from the library. A little olive or unrefined peanut oil rubbed into the skin will enliven it, and benefit those body parts lying beneath the skin too.

EXERCISE YOUR WHOLE BODY

Exercise or physical activity is just as important as proper eating and sleeping. Benefits of exercise such as improved circulation, deeper sleep, increased appetite for wholesome food, better elimination, and stronger immunity would require years to accomplish any other way. We all know how important exercise is. It's just a matter of making a routine of it.

Almost all of us get some exercise each day. Perhaps you feel this is enough for you, and are getting ready to skip ahead. If you walk for at least thirty minutes, preferably two times per day (making sixty minutes total); do some light stretching exercise, maybe fifteen minutes worth; and practice ten minutes of deep breathing, you have my permission to skip this section.

I am assuming that those of you who are reading further are not satisfied with your present efforts and would like to learn how to begin a sensible, but moderate, exercise program. It's really quite simple. First, choose a date to begin, say this coming Friday. Then decide how you want to begin. One person may choose bicycling, another swimming, a third jumping rope. Like me, you may just choose to take a long walk. Once you decide on the mode you can figure out whether it would be best to exercise before dinner or after. If you are starved at dinner time, just home from a long day, you may want to eat. On the other hand, if you don't feel you have earned your next meal, activity-wise, you may elect to exercise before dinner.

Even light exercise, when practiced regularly, will help you to better assimilate your food, lose weight, reduce nervous tension, and even solve problems. All of us have problems that need solving, and what better way to do so then to "walk" on them? Would you rather sleep on them? Imagine waking in the morning after solving problems all night!

I will close this discussion by revealing a secret that only regular exercisers know: exercise is fun. You may feel that it's not for you right now, but if you keep at it, I guarantee, you will learn my secret in a short time; and like me you will probably want to pass it on to a friend.

5

The Hippocrates Diet

The Hippocrates Diet is a natural diet. It consists of food as it is found in nature—unprocessed and unchanged. Food that will build and nourish the muscles, skin, lungs, blood, brain, nerves, and bones of your body. Food that is "living," containing a full spectrum of nutrients and enzyme activity. Food which tends to prevent health problems, aids in the body's natural healing process, promotes mental clarity, balanced body weight, and extends the span of life to its full potential.

There is much historical evidence to show that mankind first evolved in a climate that supported his every need. Without weapons for killing and fire for cooking, man lived mainly on the fruits, leaves, shoots, roots, seeds, and nuts that were abundant. He shared these with the local representatives of the animal kingdom. Only thousands of years later did man begin to move north, and having discovered fire, cook his food. Since then, and for thousands of years, we have cooked food, and although cooking methods do not always totally destroy the food enzyme value, our health has continued to decline as a result.

Since the simple hearth of the original cave-dwelling humans—whose cooked food was often eaten half raw—we have come a long way. Microwave ovens, high temperature food processing, electric cookers, deep fryers, steamers, and broilers are the modern means of destroying food enzymes and vitamins. Radiation, another modern technological development, is highly touted by the Army, and is now being considered by major food purveyors for widespread application to fresh produce, uncooked meats, milk, cheese, eggs, whole grains, seeds and beans, and all otherwise fresh foods sold in supermarkets. This process involves preserving food with dangerous rays (up to 4.5 rays of gamma radiation—10,000 times the dosage lethal to humans) and results in wholesale destruction of all the enzymes and vital properties contained in our foods.

Efficient cooking methods and an almost all-cooked diet have resulted in widespread enzyme deficiencies in modern people. After years of eating cooked, low-quality protein and enzymeless, refined carbohydrates, pancreatic breakdown and pituitary imbalance are likely. All of us can use the pancreatic support from predigested, enzyme-rich, and high-quality raw proteins and carbohydrates. On the Hippocrates Diet, which supplies these nutrients in an assimilable form, you will need less food and still get more protein and other vital nutrients. This may seem odd, but it's true—by eating less, you get more. It's not so strange when you understand that you assimilate more by improving the quality of the food you eat.

Raw, living food provides high-quality nourishment. We are all aware of the vitamin and mineral value of uncooked fruits and vegetables, but most of us are unaware that raw food has much more to offer—vital food enzymes. The food enzymes in raw food predigest the food in our stomachs, which, as discussed earlier, is the key to a long, healthy life without disease. Because of the destruction of 100 percent of the enzymes in food by cooking, and the ease of digestion of almost all raw foods, all the calories in Hippocrates diet are supplied by uncooked food.

Protein is a vital element found in abundance in the Hippocrates Diet. In earlier chapters I have pointed out the dangers of eating low-quality protein foods such as red meat. The protein foods that Americans most often consume contain large quantities of fat, are eaten cooked (which damages up to 70 percent of their available protein), and create huge amounts of waste due to their inefficient utilization by the body. On the other hand, the high-quality protein foods that we will discuss in this chapter—seeds, grains, nuts, greens, and fermented foods, are both easily and efficiently used by the body because they are eaten raw and undamaged, and do not contain excessive fats. (The fats these foods do contain are cholesterol-free, polyunsaturated fats.) Moreover, raw plant proteins produce comparatively little waste. In essence, they are the highest-quality, safest, and most efficient proteins you can eat. Even so, I do not expect you to make the change from cooked to living food overnight.

My own transition to a living foods diet took many years of experimentation, and I must admit that I am still learning. It might be helpful to set a goal for yourself over the next few weeks or months to gradually increase the amount of uncooked foods you use. In the meantime, you will make great strides forward if you can muster up the courage to empty your shelves of processed and refined items, or any others of questionable value, and replace only the necessities with natural and whole food substitutes. Don't worry about variety; there are over 150 new and tasty foods to choose from.

OVER 150 FOODS TO CHOOSE FROM

There are over 150 foods to choose from in the Hippocrates Diet. Each one contains a full spectrum of nutrients to aid their own digestion, assimilation, and elimination from your body. Enzymeless cooked foods either strain digestion and exit the body partially unassimilated, or are over-assimilated, causing you to become fat. Foods refined of their fiber can stick to your insides like glue, whereas unprocessed foods are digested, assimilated, and eliminated from your body with ease. Only what is needed is taken and body weight is normalized.

The basic food groups in the Hippocrates Diet are: fruits; vegetables and greens; fresh fruit and chlorophyll juices; sprouted seeds, grains and legumes; nuts and seeds; fermented foods; and small amounts of raw honey.

FRUITS

Fresh fruits are on the average more than 90 percent liquid, and they contain an abundance of oxygen and acids. The mild acids that fruits contain dissolve unwholesome substances, cleanse tissues, and stimulate metabolism in the human body. Have you ever eaten too much fruit or drunk too many cups of apple cider and found yourself running to the bathroom all day? Fruit does stir up things inside of us, especially if you are not used to eating a lot of it.

In the Hippocrates Diet, two to five pieces of fresh fruit can be eaten per day. If you are allergic to fresh fruits, the disturbance from the fruit enzymes is usually due to the over-acid nature of your blood and body. If you would like to try to change this condition, the book *Enzyme Nutrition,* by Dr. Edward Howell, offers a suggestion. Begin by eating one strawberry (for example) a day, and slowly increase the frequency until the fruit can be taken several times daily. Then slowly increase the quantity until you can use moderate amounts at a time. If you are prone to blood sugar imbalances such as hypoglycemia, be forewarned that you may react to fruit sugar in the same way as to cane sugar. If so, it is best to avoid sweet fruits such as raisins and figs.

If you are trying to lose weight, bananas may be your best friend. Try loading up on them occasionally, instead of eating other meals. Contrary to popular belief, although bananas are sweet, they are not fattening. Have you ever seen an obese monkey? Eat as many bananas as you like, providing the sugar doesn't affect you adversely. For that matter, eat or drink as many of the fresh juices, salads, sprouts, vegetables, sprouted grain breads, and seed and nut dishes as you like, too, and you will still lose weight. The key is raw calories from uncooked food. So go ahead, have an avocado, mango, coconut, or whatever else suits your fancy. Do you like ice cream? Have I got a recipe for you—banana ice cream (p. 144). It's so good you won't be able to tell the difference from the commercial product.

The fruits that you can use in the Hippocrates Diet are listed below. They can be used as meals, as snacks, or as desserts, but leave at least one hour between dinner and a fruit dessert for best digestion. Breakfast is the ideal time to use fruits. They wake you up, clean your stomach of residue from previous meals, and give you energy to burn. Dried fruits are a good substitute for fresh fruits in winter when seasonal fruit is scarce. Try to find the unpasteurized and unsulfured dried fruits available at natural foods grocers. Do not use dried fruits that have been sulfured (sulfur is used as a preservative) or pasteurized, as these contain enzymeless calories that can be fattening and difficult to digest. All dried fruits should be soaked in cool water until soft. Depending on the type of fruit, this may take an hour, as for raisins, or overnight, as for prunes, figs, pears, peaches, and apricots. Use enough water to cover all the fruits. After using water to soak dried fruit, you may either drink it or use it as a sweetener in recipes.

Recommended Fruits

apples
apricots—fresh and dried (unsulfured)
avocados
bananas
blackberries
blueberries
canary melon
cantaloupe
cherimoya
cherries
cranberries
crenshaw melon
currants—dried (unsulfured)
figs—fresh and dried (unsulfured)
gooseberries
grapefruits
grapes
guavas
honeydew melon
kumquats
lemons
limes
mangoes
muskmelon
nectarines
oranges
papayas
peaches
pears
Persian melon
persimmons
pineapples
plums
pomegranates
prunes—dried (unsulfured)
raisins—dried (unsulfured)
raspberries
strawberries
tangerines
watermelon

VEGETABLES AND GREENS

All vegetables cultivated by humans were once herbs that grew wild. After years of experimentation, we have our common garden vegetables of today. Vegetables, including salad greens, contain valuable organic mineral elements and vitamins. Their mineral salts neutralize and help eliminate systemic waste from the body.

They are also a good source of natural fiber that gives the muscles in the colon a good workout. Each day eat as much raw salad as you like. Use greens, sprouts, an assortment of vegetables, and other ingredients such as seeds, nuts, and avocados. Use plenty of green vegetables and leafy greens each day to supply the necessary calcium and iron salts, but be sure to include a variety of different colored vegetables, sprouts, and dressings each day to ensure adequate vitamin intake.

It should take you at least twenty to thirty minutes to polish off a salad that satisfies you. In colder weather you can warm the ingredients to room temperature after taking from the refrigerator. This can be done merely by setting them out for a time before eating, or by placing the vegetables in a heat-resistant bowl in an open pot of boiling water for a minute or so. Cold salad could make you feel cold.

Recommended Vegetables and Greens

alfalfa (fresh)
alfalfa sprouts
artichokes (Jerusalem)
asparagus
bean sprouts (all types)
beans (fresh)
beets
beet greens
bok choy
Brussels sprouts
buckwheat greens
cabbage (green or red)
cabbage, sprouted
carrots
cauliflower
celery
Chinese cabbage
chives
collards
comfrey leaves
corn on the cob
cucumbers
dandelion greens
dill
endive
escarole
fenugreek sprouts
garlic
green beans
green peas (edible pod)
green peppers
kale
kohlrabi
lamb's-quarters
leeks
lettuce (all types)
mung bean sprouts
mushrooms
mustard greens
okra

onions
parsley
parsnips
potatoes
purslane
radish sprouts
radishes
red peppers
scallions
shallots
spinach
squash—soft summer varieties
sunflower greens
Swiss chard
tomatoes
turnips
turnip greens
yams
yellow wax beans
watercress
wheatgrass

Be sure to try greens, green herbs, and green vegetables you have never used before. You may find some pleasant surprises. After you have been eating green foods for six months to one year, you will feel that something is missing unless you have them each day. When you recognize this, your body is beginning to take a more active role in food selection, and that is the purpose of any good health program—to help you tune in to your own body's needs. There are many chlorophyll-rich foods which can be juiced or eaten in salads. Don't worry, you won't turn green!

FRESH JUICES FROM FRUITS AND VEGETABLES

Fresh juices, extracted from fruits, sprouts, and vegetables, are a valuable component of the Hippocrates Diet. They are packed with vitamins, minerals, food enzymes, amino acids, and natural sugars that provide raw calories, and are easily assimilated by the body. Fresh juices also supply valuable electrolytes and oxygen to the cells of the body for use in cleansing and rebuilding. Above all, they taste great!

Natural beverages such as fresh fruit juices, green drinks, Rejuvelac, and seed milks replace all carbonated and artificially sweetened beverages, coffee, tea, and milk on the Hippocrates Diet. Since bottled fruit juices and juices sold in cartons at the supermarket are almost always pasteurized, they are not recommended. Instead, any of these juices that you like can be used fresh. That is, you should run whole apples (without the seeds) through your juicer, or squeeze oranges yourself at home.

Use at least two glasses of fresh mixed green juices each day. Strain out the pulp to improve the flavor and make the juices easier to digest. One eight-ounce glass a half hour or so before lunch and one before dinner, or one before dinner and before bed, will supply one pint, which is about the amount you should have each day. Use vegetable juice rather than fruit juice an hour before bed. While you sleep, it will work to aid elimination.

Chlorophyll Juices

Chlorophyll is the pigment that gives trees, grasses, and leafy plants their characteristic green color. More importantly, chlorophyll enables plants to convert the energy of the sun into nutrients that can be utilized by living things.

Chlorophyll-rich plant juices supply rich land-based minerals and chlorophyll proteins to Hippocrates dieters. Fresh chlorophyll juices from greens and herbs such as parsley or watercress are also rich in vitamins. Ideally, these should be juiced in a slow-turning juicer and used fresh every day.

Iron is another key factor in the green plants used as food in the Hippocrates Diet. Without sufficient iron from green foods, there is a possibility that you could suffer from anemia. Although this is unlikely if you follow a balanced diet, fresh green juices will safeguard against it. Juicing enables us to capture the micronutrients of several pounds of vegetables in a single glass. Unlike concentrated vitamin-mineral supplements, fresh juices are non-toxic in any amount. In fact, there is evidence that the properties of green juices can protect us from radiation, smoke inhalation, and all forms of pollution, draw toxic metals like lead, cadmium, and mercury out of the system, and even prevent cancer. The best sources for green juices are listed below. In addition, vegetables which are not green, such as carrots, tomatoes, and summer squashes, may be used as flavoring.

Sources of Green Juices

- alfalfa (fresh)
- alfalfa sprouts
- bean sprouts (all types)
- beet greens
- bok choy
- buckwheat greens
- cabbage
- cabbage sprouts
- celery
- Chinese cabbage
- chives
- collards
- comfrey leaves
- cucumbers
- dandelion greens
- green (snap) beans
- green peppers
- kale
- lamb's-quarters
- lettuce (all types)
- parsley
- purslane
- scallions
- spinach
- sunflower greens
- Swiss chard
- turnip greens
- wheatgrass
- watercress

SEA VEGETABLES

I bet you never thought you would ever eat those stringy bits of multi-colored seaweed you come across as you walk along the beach. I didn't, either, until I learned about their remarkable nutritional contents. For me to actually taste them was a giant step. Yet I have come to depend on them to supply some of the minerals and nutrients that have been leached from inorganically fertilized modern topsoil.

As plants grow, they convert dissolved inorganic mineral compounds into organic mineral salts that are more easily used by humans. The abundance of minerals and trace elements in ocean water and on the ocean floor makes sea vegetables particularly valuable in our diet. Sea vegetables such as dulse, kelp, arame, nori, wakame, kombu, or hiziki, should be used each day. Dulse and kelp are frequently available in powdered form. Two tablespoons total is plenty. As a group, the sea vegetables are one of the richest food sources of minerals and trace elements.

Dr. Weston Price, in his travels to Peru, noticed natives of the Andes Mountains carrying a little bag around with them wherever they went. The bag contained kelp from the Peruvian coast, more than a month's journey from the natives' home. When asked why they carried it, the Indians replied, "It guards the heart." The presence of sea vegetables in the diet may also prevent baldness and enhance vitality.

Historically, the coastal Japanese, Irish, Canadians, American Indians, and many other cultures have used sea vegetables as a regular item in their diets. In fact, a snack food made from dulse, a purple sea vegetable harvested off the Atlantic coasts of the U.S., Canada, and the British Isles, was once sold by street vendors in Boston and is still served in pubs in Scotland, Ireland, and Canada. The Japanese eat dozens of varieties of fresh and dried sea vegetables. The Russians sell "sea cabbage"—canned sea vegetables mixed with garden vegetables. They also make a type of whiskey from a reddish-colored sea vegetable. By eating sea vegetables, these various peoples are assured of getting a full range of minerals and trace elements such as boron, selenium, iodine, calcium, potassium, magnesium, iron, and others that are not always found in necessary quantities in ordinary garden vegetables. These traditional sea vegetable foods are not recommended for use in the Hippocrates Diet, however, because they are cooked (depleted of enzymes) or alcoholic (toxic). Fresh or dried sea vegetables are most beneficial when they're uncooked and unprocessed.

The two sea vegetables that figure most prominently in the Hippocrates Diet are kelp and dulse. Both of them give food a slightly salty flavor—they contain a percentage of sea salt, which is rich in minerals. The Japanese grade seaweeds according to cleanliness, taste, freshness, tenderness, size and appearance, and by paying attention to these classifications, you may be assured of the quality of the sea vegetables you purchase.

The name kelp covers a wide variety of sea vegetables, mostly dark green in color. Kelp grows in abundance off the California coast and is available at most natural foods stores. The Hippocrates Diet uses kelp powder added to dressings and seed ferments, or sprinkled on salads.

Dulse is popular at the Institute. It is eaten as a snack food with a piece of celery or carrot, and used in preparing live food meals. Both kelp and dulse are pleasant additions to soups.

As the other sea vegetables that are part of the Hippocrates Diet may be unfamiliar to you, they deserve a few words by way of identification. Arame and hiziki are dark-colored spaghetti-like sea vegetables available at most natural foods stores. They can be added to salads, dressings, and breads, or made into sea vegetable salads (see Recipes for ideas). Nori is the dried sheets of the dark-colored sea vegetable used to make the sushi rolls commonly served at Japanese restaurants. On the Hippocrates Diet, sushi rolls can be used to wrap anything from sprout salads to cauliflower loaves. For best results, get an inexpensive bamboo sushi roller and use it to make perfect live food sushi every time. The green-colored sea vegetables kombu and wakame are too tough for general use unless they are eaten in small quantities, finely chopped or powdered.

Sea vegetables should be soaked in enough warm (not hot) water to cover, for 10–20 minutes or until they are soft enough to slice. The time will vary—dulse, arame, hiziki, and nori take just a few minutes to soften up, whereas wakame and kombu are tougher. Always discard the soaking water from sea water used to soak sea vegetables, because it has an extremely high sodium (salt) content.

Selected Sea Vegetables

arame
dulse
hiziki
kelp
kombu
nori
wakame

SPROUTED SEEDS, GRAINS, AND LEGUMES

All seeds, beans, and grains contain enzyme inhibitors to preserve their contents until the proper environmental conditions awaken them to life. If these foods are eaten unsoaked or unsprouted the inhibitors can intefere with your digestion and assimilation of their nutrients.

Sprouts

Sprouts are a highly nutritious, easily used, easily digested, and inexpensive food. By growing your own you can have a year-round supply of fresh food for only pennies a serving. Sprouting transforms the nutrients of seeds, grains, and beans into easily digested, high-energy foods, similar to vegetables, but more concentrated in nutrients. Use a variety of sprouts each day in your salads.

Recommended Sprouts

adzuki
alfalfa
almond
cabbage
chick pea
clover
corn
cow pea
fenugreek
green pea
lentil
millet
mung
mustard
oats
radish
rye
sesame
soybean
sunflower
triticale
watercress
wheat

Grains and Breads

Sprouted grains can also be used in breads. Breads have been a staple food for all peoples for centuries. Our ancestors always soaked their grain before baking bread. This removed the enzyme inhibitors and brought the grain to life. The center of the bread often remained raw with food enzymes intact. Most of today's bread is made from bleached white flour with added chemicals, and is overcooked. It has little or no natural food value and certainly no food enzymes.

Whole wheat or sourdough breads made from whole grains are a vast improvement over white bread, but are still deficient in enzymes. For a bread to be truly healthful, it is best made from sprouted grain which has been dried in the sun or in a dehydrator. Sprouted grain bread and crisps are essential to the Hippocrates Diet. They supply calories and are a good source of complex carbohydrates, high-quality proteins, and minerals. Try making breads in several different ways until you get the one you like just right.

Sprouting grain and blending or mixing it with fruits or other foods is another good way to eat it. For example, blended with some warm water and raisins, sprouted wheat makes a great breakfast with a lot of "fire power" to get you through a long day.

Legumes

Legumes (beans and peas) are among the oldest foods known to man. For thousands of years, they have provided us with valuable proteins and mineral salts. They can be thought of as natural fertilizers for the body, enriching it with earthy nutrients. The protein they yield is high-quality and easily assimilated. Dr. Jeffrey Bland, a professor of nutritional biochemistry at the University of Puget Sound in Washington, found that six cups of lentil sprouts fulfilled the complete protein needs of an adult male for an entire day, providing more than fifty grams of protein.

There are many varieties of edible legumes available in the United States. Especially good are sprouted adzuki, mung beans, lentil beans, cow peas, and chick peas. Soybeans are unpalatable unless made into a milk, and should only be used on occasion, if at all. The other beans can be used as often as you desire, as long as they are sprouted first.

NUTS AND SEEDS

Raw nuts and seeds are a prime source of body-building protein. When sprouted, their enzyme inhibitors are neutralized, and they become a rich source of raw calories. An overnight soaking will also neutralize their enzyme inhibitors. To soak seeds or nuts, hull or shell them and place them in a bowl with spring or filtered water. Use more than enough water to cover them, because they will swell up. Always discard the water used to soak seeds and nuts, because of its chemical content.

Use a portion of germinated nuts and seeds at each meal in salads, sauces, dressings, loaves, and so on. Ten to twenty almonds (soaked) are a good quantity for a portion; have more if few other sprouts are being used. The list of wonderful and appetizing foods you can make with seeds and nuts is endless. Shakes, yogurts, cheeses, dressings, milks, trail mix, fruit creams, and ice creams are just a few. How would you like to try my Lemon Mayonnaise Dressing, or Almond Frappé with banana ice cream?

Recommended Nuts and Seeds

almonds
Brazil nuts
coconuts
hazel nuts
(filberts)
pecans
pine nuts
pumpkin seeds
sesame seeds
squash seeds
sunflower seeds
walnuts

FERMENTED AND PREDIGESTED FOODS

Fermentation is the decomposition or acidification of organic substances produced by the action of living organisms—enzymes. During the fermentation process, proteins, starches, and fats in foods are broken up into more simple compounds. Foods that have been broken up by enzymes outside of the body are called predigested foods. Sauerkraut, pickles and pickled vegetables, seed yogurt, miso (a fermented soybean paste), seed or nut cheese, sourdough, sprouted (raw) bread, and Rejuvelac are examples of predigested foods in the Hippocrates Diet. Other foods like fruits, some sprouts, and honey are predigested (ripened) by nature. As a rule, predigested foods require less enzyme output and digestive work than more complex or cooked foods.

The use of fermented foods, along with abstinence from meats and refined foods, will turn the unhealthy alkaline condition of the colon into a healthy acid one. Dr. Metchnikoff, a longevity researcher at the Pasteur Institute, found this alkaline condition of the colon—brought on by the use of meat and other animal foods and subsequent autointoxication of the colon and body—to be the main reason why we die so young. He advocated the use of fermented foods and abstinence from meat and refined foods to restore an acid condition to the bowel.

You may use fermented foods as often as you like, as long as you eat foods from the other categories recommended in Chapter 1.

HONEY

Raw honey is a good source of calories, energy, some vitamins, minerals, and food enzymes. In addition it is easily digested, requiring little aid from the body. Dark honeys like buckwheat, rice, or wildflower honey, contain more minerals than lighter varieties. All honey should be purchased raw and unfiltered. The raw honey may crystallize on the shelf of the store or at home. Put it in warm water (not boiling) to liquefy it again. Honey can be used in Rejuvelac, lemon water, fruit sauces, raw candies, or other dishes. Try to limit quantity to one or two tablespoons per day or less.

TRANSITION

Now that I have described what the Hippocrates Diet is made up of, here comes the important part—what it isn't made up of. More than 20,000 processed items available on supermarket shelves are banned, including commercial ice cream, bonbons, and white flour. Beef, pork, chicken, eggs, dairy products, and fast foods are also prohibited. Ideally, cooked foods should be minimized or avoided altogether.

What will you eat? Make it a point to clear your shelves of refined, foodless foods and replace them with natural substitutes.

Hippocrates Diet Foods, Transitional Foods, and Items to Avoid

Food Category	Hippocrates Diet Foods
Proteins	fermented seed and nut sauces, yogurts, and cheeses; seed milks; sprouted seeds, beans, and nuts; avocados; green drinks
Carbohydrates	grain crisps; sprouted grain breads, cereals, and warmed cereals; sprouted wheat loaves; grain milks; sprouted pie crusts; treats
Fats/Oils	avocados; seed and nut cheeses; fresh raw nut butters in small amounts; vegetable and seed yogurt dressings
Vegetables	uncooked sprouts and greens; organically grown; pickled with no salt; dried, blended into soups or sauces; juiced
Fruits	*fresh*: sauces, soups, salads, shakes, milks, pies, banana ice cream; *dried, unsulfured*: snacks, raw candies
Beverages	Rejuvelac; fresh fruit and vegetable juices; spring or distilled water; green drinks
Snacks	vegetable sticks; fresh fruit; sprouted trail mix; grain crisps; fresh juice; dried fruit and nut candies; seed cheese on celery sticks
Condiments	raw unfiltered honey; bee pollen; fresh fruits; dried fruits; miso; tamari; veggie salt; kelp powder; sauerkraut; lemons, lemon juice; fresh and dried herbs

Transitional Foods	Avoid Altogether
slow-cooked beans and peas (soups); tofu; tempeh; nut butters; unsoaked nuts and seeds	red meats; fish; poultry; eggs; pasteurized milk and cheeses; hydrolized vegetable proteins; luncheon meats; meat analogs
sourdough breads (no yeast); unleavened crackers; whole slow-cooked rice, wheat, millet, buckwheat, barley, oats, cornmeal, bulghur, rye; sprouted grain breads; natural granola	all yeasted breads and flour products; processed grains; white rice; noodles, pasta; granola with sugar; baked goods containing refined oils; sugar; refined flour; additives
small amounts of unrefined sesame or olive oil on salads; nut butters; sesame tahini	all oils except sesame and olive; commercial nut butters; peanuts; pasteurized butter or cream; all foods containing or cooked in oils
steamed (no oil); slow-baked; soups and stews; broth; en casserole; inorganically grown	frozen; irradiated; canned; overcooked; cooked with sugar and/ or salt; stale or wilted; pickled with salt
cooked fruits or cooked fruit desserts; baked apples; soaked and steamed dried fruits; steamed fruits; apple sauce	canned or preserved with chemicals and added sugar; sulfured dried; unripe
bottled natural fruit and vegetable juices; herb teas; natural carbonated drinks; grain coffee	tap water; coffee; tea; soda; alcoholic drinks; artificially sweetened fruit drinks
rice cakes; natural granola; unleavened crackers; trail mix; rice sushi; baked apples; bottled juices; popcorn (no oil or butter); herb tea; grain coffee; rice syrup candy	natural and unnatural junk food snacks; commercial "health" food snacks; soda; candies
pasteurized honey; maple syrup; barley malt; rice syrup; sorghum; cider vinegar; sea salt; garlic; onion; cayenne; chili spices; powdered vegetable enzymes; natural cooking wine	*products containing additives, including*: sugar, molasses, cane syrup, dextrose (glucose), fructose, salt, iodized salt, vinegar, pepper, monosodium glutamate (MSG), oils, eggs, coloring, and preservatives

Sample as many whole, local, and fresh foods as possible. And if you have a choice of eating something raw or cooked, eat it raw. Reduce the amount of cooking you do to a minimum, satisfying your craving for hot foods with uncooked, but warmed, soups or cereals.

Other transition ideas are to eat whole foods whenever possible, avoiding flour-based and processed items. Whole foods are foods that are eaten just as they are found in nature. Some examples are: brown rice as opposed to milled white rice; whole wheat as opposed to white flour products; and baked potatoes with the skin, instead of mashed potatoes. Most natural foods stores specialize in selling bulk and packaged whole grains, beans, seeds, nuts, vegetables, and fruits.

If you consume mostly live and whole foods you will be eating a diet which is low in fats, adequate in protein, and high in energy-producing complex carbohydrates. Even after cooking, foods like vegetables, beans, brown rice, and other whole grains, are superior to high-fat, high-protein and energy-poor red meats, poultry, milk, eggs, cheese, fish, and so on.

These suggestions are especially helpful for those people who desire a gradual changeover to the Hippocrates Diet. In addition, I strongly urge anyone who is serious about improving and maintaining his health to visit our Institute for a two-week course.

WHAT WILL YOU EAT?

The most nutritious things you can eat are the fresh foods that are sold at natural foods groceries and supermarkets and the super-nutritious foods you can grow yourself at home—greens, sprouts, and wheatgrass. Even if you live in a big city, on the tenth floor, you can still grow plenty of nutritious food. The next two chapters will tell you how.

So—what will you eat? Whether you plunge right into a living foods diet and home gardening, or choose to adapt to the Hippocrates Diet more gradually, the following chart will be a useful guide. The chart on pages 54–55 has three main groupings: (1) the Hippocrates Diet foods, (2) transitional foods, which I suggest be used moderately as a flavoring for the Hippocrates Diet group, and (3) many popular foods that I suggest you avoid altogether. The first part of the chart presents the various foods that comprise our diet in terms of nutritional composition: proteins, carbohydrates, and fats/oils. The lower portion of the chart lists the food categories that round out our diet: vegetables, fruits, beverages, snacks, and condiments. The methods of preparing specific foods, both preferred and prohibited, are indicated.

6

Indoor Gardening For Beginners

To grow food for a family of four, living in a city environment, you don't have to spread soil on top of your carpet or plant an apple tree in your bathtub! In this and the next chapter, I am going to discuss some simple gardening techniques that require a minimum of time and effort yet can yield a tremendous quantity of high-quality nutrition for you and your family, all year long. There are basically two types of foods you can grow indoors simply and with little effort. One group, greens and grass, is the subject of this chapter. The other group of indoor garden foods is sprouts, which are covered in the next chapter.

Freshly grown buckwheat lettuce, sunflower greens, and wheatgrass are a tasty and nutritious addition to any really healthful diet. Grown on an inch of soil in just seven days, they can replace more expensive lettuce and salad greens.

Pound for pound, sprouts and indoor garden greens are the least expensive foods for the amount of nutrition they supply. For example, one pound of alfalfa seed, which retails for around three dollars, yields eight pounds of high-quality nutrition when sprouted. That's 37 cents per pound. And at anywhere from 13 to 24 cents per pound (that is what it will cost you to grow it) wheatgrass can save you plenty of money, too.

There is nothing difficult about growing your own fresh salad greens at home. At the Hippocrates Institute we have created an indoor gardening system for growing buckwheat lettuce, sunflower greens, and wheatgrass. Indoor gardening requires little time and effort—and no costly supplies. In fact, a juicer for the purpose of juicing wheatgrass, sprouts, and greens is about the only item you may want to send away for. The rest of the supplies are inexpensive and can be found locally. (If you prefer, these are also available by mail. See the Appendix.)

For the past seven years, I have been growing enough food in my tiny third-floor apartment kitchen to feed a small army. I go to the trouble of growing a good portion of my food to guarantee its cleansing properties, safety, and nutritional value. In addition, there are land use, economic, and quality considerations.

It takes nearly ten times more land to produce as much protein in meat form as the equivalent in plant foods. Cattle farming wastes millions of acres of land where nut trees, vegetables, seeds, and grains could be grown to supply all the world's people with adequate nutrition. A leading proponent of vegetarianism, Frances Moore Lappé, author of *Diet for A Small Planet*, points out that eating meat to get protein is about as efficient as paddling a canoe with a chopstick. It takes over twenty pounds of grain to add one pound of beef to the human feedlot.

One more reason to grow food indoors is quality assurance. At home you can produce fresh food that you know has not been tampered with. No chemicals have been used to grow it. No gasses have been used to ripen or refrigerate it. And no additives have been put in to preserve it during shipping and distribution. The food you grow is fresh when you want it, whereas store-bought produce may be several days old by the time you get it. Sprouts and garden greens are still growing even after you harvest them. The only problem this could create would be that a sprout loaf left over from dinner one night could double in size by the next night when you went to use it!

Seriously, though, indoor gardening can give you a certain amount of control over your food supply with a minimum of effort. Young green plants have a few simple needs: sun, water, a little soil, and proper growing temperature. Plants know how to capture the sun, mix it with the air and water, reinforce it with minerals from the soil, and grow. You don't have to be a long-time organic gardener or have a green thumb to grow perfect greens and sprouts every time.

SETTING UP AN INDOOR GARDEN

The first step in setting up your own indoor garden system will be finding a location to plant and store the trays of greens. You will also need a place to keep seeds and topsoil or compost. Since I live on the third floor of our Boston Institute, I both plant and store all my supplies right in my kitchen. If you own a house you may want to set up the system in your basement, garage, or on the back porch, or, as I have done, in your kitchen. You may also choose to break up the operations, for example, by storing soil and actually planting in the basement, setting the trays in the upstairs windows, and soaking your seeds in jars by the kitchen sink. Whatever setup you choose, though, you will need plenty of indirect sunlight for the growing plants and a warm place to start the trays off during the winter months (65–75° F is ideal).

If the thought of bringing soil into your home bothers you, and you have no place to grow things outdoors, don't panic. Although there is no real substitute for fresh greens and wheatgrass grown on good soil, there are ways to grow both without soil in automatic sprouters. I use one of these to grow my sprouts at home, but I still prefer to use soil to grow greens and wheatgrass. This is because after five days of growth the young plants begin to look for nutrients not found in the seed, but found in the soil. Thus, for two to five days the greens and wheatgrass grown in automatic sprouting machines are in need of outside nutrients that are not available. The result is food and green juice which aren't as potent as they could be. However, if soilless growing is the only way you can foresee growing and using buckwheat lettuce, sunflower greens, and wheatgrass, it is far better than having none at all.

To grow greens and wheatgrass in your automatic sprouter follow the sprouting instructions in Chapter 7, using unhulled buckwheat and sunflower seeds. Grow both the wheatgrass and greens an extra two to five days in the unit.

GROWING INDOOR GREENS AND WHEATGRASS ON SOIL

If you use the method that I recommend, you will need to seek out some good topsoil and some peat moss, or a mixture of topsoil and compost (I will discuss compost in more detail at the end of this chapter). Topsoil is the first twelve to twenty inches of dark-colored soil immediately beneath the grass on your lawn, or under the leaves covering the surface of a wooded area. If you live in a city, rather than risk being jailed for digging in the park, get some topsoil from a friend in the suburbs, or buy a few large bags from a garden supply store.

When taking topsoil from a wooded area, especially where pine trees are growing, mix about a half pint of ground limestone (lime) into a trash barrel full of soil. This will offset the acidity of the soil and make your wheatgrass richer-tasting and easier to grow. Lime is inexpensive, and is available at any garden center. Ordinary lawn topsoil does not usually need lime, but you can add a handful or two per barrelful of soil just to be on the safe side. If you aren't mixing compost into the soil, mix it with peat moss, also available at garden shops, in a fifty-fifty ratio. If you are using compost from an outdoor garden, it should be screened before being mixed with the topsoil, to remove large stones, sticks, and other debris.

To produce one tray of greens and another of wheatgrass per day you will need to start off with at least two barrels full of topsoil and half a bale of peat moss. Along with this you will need two additional empty barrels to begin composting the used plant mats. Four barrels, two of which are filled with soil, and a half bale of peat moss will take care of your soil needs for a few weeks. After that time you will be able to use the recycled soil mats from the compost barrels.

For planting the seeds and wheat, I recommend that you purchase some hard plastic trays. Restaurant supply stores will often sell you cafeteria trays about 10" × 14" in size. Of these you will need one to hold the soil and another to cover each planted tray for the first three days. So in all you will need about fifteen trays if you plan to have a tray per day of each.

To soak your wheat, or sunflower and buckwheat seeds, you will need some wide-mouth jars. While seeds are soaking and sprouting cover the jars with squares of nylon mesh and a rubber band (as described in the chapter on sprouting). Try to get strong rubber bands, as weak ones can snap and the sprouts will go everywhere.

Besides water and a little patience, the only other thing you will need is seed. "Hard" or "winter" wheatberries are the ones we use to grow wheatgrass. If possible, obtain organically grown seeds from a natural food store. Sprays and fertilizers lodged in plant fibers are toxic and sprayed seeds do not grow or sprout well. When purchasing buckwheat or sunflower seeds to grow for greens buy them with their hulls on, or "unhulled." The amount of wheatberries and seed to use per tray will vary according to the size of tray you're using, but in general one cup of dry wheatberries will be the right amount for a 10" × 14" tray. For the greens, three-quarters cup of sunflower and one-half cup of buckwheat will do.

Planting Instructions

Before planting, wash seeds to remove any grime or dust. Next, place them in the jar and fill it with water. Put a screen over the top and let it sit overnight (or for twelve hours). Drain the wheat after soaking, rinse it well and let it sprout in the jar at a 45° angle, for another twelve hours—making twenty-four hours from the time you washed the seed to the time of planting.

Now spread a layer of soil one inch deep at the bottom of the tray, leaving small trenches around the edges to catch excess water, and smooth it out. Pour the sprouted wheat or seeds in the middle of the tray and spread them out evenly with your hands, covering the soil. Ideally, one seed should touch another on all sides, but should not have any others piled on top of it. Sprinkle the tray with water, making it damp (but not swampy), and cover with another tray. The second tray, used as a cover, acts as a mini-greenhouse which keeps moisture and heat in, and light out, of the growing environment. After you have watered and covered the tray, set it aside for three days.

At the end of three days uncover the tray, water it well, and place it in indirect light. The more light the plants get the larger and thicker the leaves and blades of grass will be. Too little light will produce tall, leggy plants with tiny leaves. A good balance of indirect sunlight and shade will produce thick, green, and juicy greens and wheatgrass.

If you uncover a tray and see a bunch of greenish-blue mold instead of baby plants, you may have had bad seeds or you may have drowned them by oversoaking. It is also possible that you may have over-watered the tray after planting. Next time try new seed, less water, and make sure that the spot where you put the tray is not too warm. It should be between 65–75° F.

Once the greens or wheatgrass are set out in the light, they will need to be watered every day or every other day depending on the weather, humidity and indoor temperature. The first or second time you water the plants, mix in a tablespoon of powdered kelp so that the plants will take up the added trace minerals and iodine. Try not to muddy the soil, but keep it moist at all times. If by accident a tray is allowed to dry out, avoid the temptation to flood it with water, as this will shock the young plants further. Moisten the soil instead, and make sure it doesn't dry out again for the next two

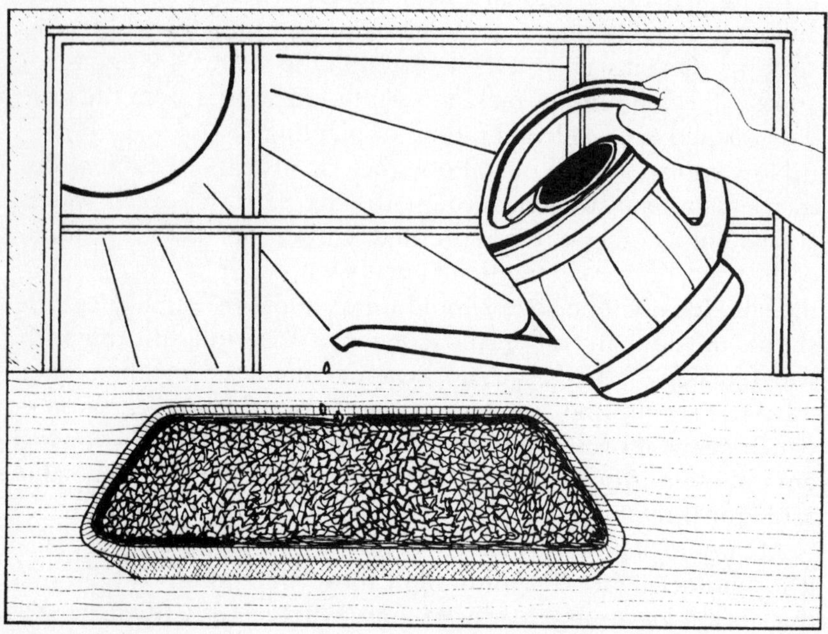

Essential Elements for Sprouting Greens: water, sunlight, soil, and warmth. Note the small trench for drainage around the edge of the tray.

days. Don't worry if the plants refuse to stand up straight again. Drooping is caused by lack of water, and the greens can be eaten anyway.

After about seven days your greens and wheatgrass will be about 7–10 inches tall and ready to harvest. In cooler weather, it may take a little longer for greens and grasses to fully mature, but during hot summer weather they can reach 10 inches in five days.

To harvest the buckwheat and sunflower greens or wheatgrass, cut as close to the soil as possible without pulling up lumps of soil with the plants. Many nutrients are concentrated close to the soil. A sharp knife and a sawing action will cut easily. If you do pull up some soil with the plants, merely rinse the root end with plain water before juicing or eating them. Do not rinse greens or grass if you are going to store them in the refrigerator, as water speeds their decomposition. Ideally, wheatgrass should be juiced and used immediately after cutting. Although cut grass can be stored for up to seven days in plastic bags in the refrigerator, once juiced it will begin to go bad in a half hour, and be completely spoiled in twelve hours.

Buckwheat and sunflower greens will last longer in the refrigerator than wheatgrass, and can be juiced any time. However, the fresher they are the better-tasting they will be, and the more nutritious as well.

Planting Instructions Checklist

As a handy reference to growing indoor garden greens and wheatgrass I have summarized the steps that we have discussed in this section.

- Mix 2–3 barrels of topsoil 50–50 with peat moss or screened compost. Obtain about 15 hard plastic cafeteria trays to use for planting and covering the planted trays, several wide-mouth jars in which to soak and sprout seeds, and seeds to plant.

- Wash the seeds and soak for 12 hours; then allow them to sprout for another 12 hours.

- Spread soil one inch deep on trays, leaving shallow trenches around the edges to catch excess water. Smooth the soil and spread the sprouted seeds on top.
- Water the planted tray, cover with another tray, and set aside for 3 days.
- On day 4, uncover the tray, water, and set in indirect light. Continue watering the tray daily or every other day, as needed, to keep it moist.
- Harvest plants with a sharp knife when they reach 7–10 inches in height, cutting as close to the roots as possible without pulling up lumps of soil. Use wheatgrass and greens as soon after harvesting as possible, and store the unused portions in a plastic bag in the refrigerator.

COMPOSTING USED GREEN AND WHEATGRASS MATS

After you have harvested your greens and wheatgrass you will be left with a mat of roots and short stems which can easily be recycled to make new soil for planting in a few weeks. This process is called composting. Compost is a mixture of ordinary topsoil and plant or animal residues which have been broken down into a rich humus by the worms, microorganisms, and enzymes in the soil.

Composting is nature's way of building, improving, and maintaining the fertility of soil. In the forest, fallen leaves and dead branches cover the earth, making rich compost for the trees that continue to grow. In fact, everything that has been taken from the soil to nourish growing plants must be returned to it through decomposition of plant and animal matter if the soil is to continue to support new growth. This is the law of nature.

Modern growing techniques used by agribusiness farmers often neglect to replace the trace elements and organic matter removed from the soil over the years. What little of these vital elements that is put back into the soil often comes in the form of synthetic chemical fertilizers. Unfortunately, there is no food in synthetic fertilizers to support soil enzymes, worms, and microorganisms that live on organic matter—and after a few years the soil becomes a useless desert, barely able to sustain weeds. Acres upon acres of land all over the world are being ruined in this way every year.

Composting is one solution to the problem of soil depletion. It is a way of reclaiming poor soil and restoring natural balance to the topsoil. Composting adds organic matter and enables soil enzymes and organisms like the friendly earthworm to thrive and multiply, enriching the soil and providing the plants grown on it with top-quality plant nutrients. This is precisely the way nature has preserved plant life on earth for centuries. And it's the only way we can ensure that the soil will be fertile enough to produce food for our children—and theirs.

An important worker in your home compost pile is the earthworm, whose job it is to digest organic matter and convert it into rich plant nutrients. Earthworm castings are an extremely valuable source of nitrogen and other minerals and nutrients. The castings that are left behind after earthworms eat and digest the soil contain five times the nitrogen, seven times the phosphate, and eleven times the potassium of ordinary topsoil.

You can obtain earthworms from a compost pile or an old pile of leaves, or you can buy some at any bait and tackle shop. Ask for red wigglers. A couple of handfuls are sufficient to get an entire colony started. Earthworms will go to work producing their weight in castings every twenty-four hours.

Composting Instructions

To get started with your home composting system you will need two empty barrels with lids, and maybe a third and fourth in time. Drill holes spaced at two-inch intervals all around the sides of the barrels. Place a shallow container of some sort under each barrel. Inverted flat trash can lids work well. It is best if this setup is supported an inch or two off the ground, to allow for air circulation underneath. A couple of bricks will do nicely.

When you have harvested some wheatgrass or greens, break up the mats into smaller pieces and place them in a layer in the bottom of the barrel. On top of this layer, spread any vegetable kitchen scraps or juicer pulp you have. Following the scraps, put in the earthworms, and cover them with another layer of broken-up mats. (Store scraps and pulp in a sealed container until you have enough mats to cover them.) As you harvest mats, repeat this layering technique, adding a handful of ground limestone instead of any more earthworms, until the barrel is full. After each layer is placed in the barrel, cover with the lid.

When the compost barrel is full, the decomposition of the mats and vegetable matter intensifies. As long as the barrels are in a warm place, but out of direct sunlight (the sun will dry them out), the compost will be ready to use in two to three months. If you want to use your compost sooner, in one to two months, remove the lid every week and stir up the contents of the barrel with a pitchfork. This will expose the inside of the barrel to more oxygen, speeding up the rate of decomposition of the contents.

You will know the compost is ready by scooping out a shovelful and examining it. If it is crumbly, dark, and without any bad odor or traces of scraps, it is ready. To use the new compost for planting, mix it with 25 percent peat moss.

Compost barrels can be kept in the basement, a back hallway, on the porch, or in a closet. Even better, purchase some attractive barrels with wheels and tight-fitting lids, and keep them right in your kitchen where they are more accessible. You don't have to worry about any unpleasant odors using this easy composting system. Properly composted earth has a pleasant, woodsy smell.

Should your compost develop an odor, it is probably because your soil mats were too wet or you did not cover kitchen scraps properly. To avoid these pitfalls, cover scraps totally with mats and avoid adding freshly watered mats to the can. Instead, let them dry out until they are moist, but not wet. If more than a few drops of moisture are collecting under the can, the compost is probably too moist. To eliminate any odor that develops, sprinkle a couple of handfuls of lime into the pile, mix it up with a pitchfork, sprinkle a few more handfuls of lime on the top layer, and cover.

Composting Instructions Checklist

The main points of my easy composting system are:

- Obtain 2 barrels and drill holes spaced 2 inches apart all around.

- Place broken-up mats at the bottom of the barrel, followed by kitchen scraps and juicer pulp, a few earthworms, and another layer of broken-up mats to cover. When you have additional mats, repeat the layers, without adding more worms, but instead adding a handful of ground limestone, until the barrel is full. Always re-cover the barrel.
- Let the full barrel sit for 2 to 3 months, at which time your compost will be ready to be mixed with 25 percent peat moss for planting. Alternatively, you can stir up the contents of the barrel each week until the compost is ready one or two months later.

If you regularly maintain an outdoor compost pile using a method without animal manures, you may add your mats to it instead. But during the winter months you will be better off if you have a ready supply of compost, and a few barrels in progress indoors, until you can put them out again in the spring. At the Hippocrates Institute we send our compost every year or two to our mini-farm in exchange for a fresh supply. The old compost is placed in the gardens, and is reconditioned by the elements. Such a rotation is ideal, as the soil will eventually need to be exposed to the air, rain and sun if it is to stay healthy and balanced.

Home-grown greens should become an important part of your diet. Combined with fresh sprouts they can supply more than 50 percent of your entire food supply. In winter especially, you should grow plenty of greens to replace expensive store-bought produce.

Should you have any further questions or problems setting up your own indoor gardening system at home, don't hesitate to call the Institute and speak to one of our experts. Better yet, come and stay for the two-week course, and learn-by-doing while you're here.

7

Super Nutrition From Sprouts

Can you imagine seeing a classified ad in the newspaper that reads:

> *$1 Million Reward* for information leading to the creation of an edible plant food that grows in any climate, rivals both beef and store-bought produce in nutritional value, matures in three to five days, may be planted any time, requires neither soil nor sunshine, equals oranges and tomatoes in Vitamin C, has no waste, can be eaten without processing or preparation, is digested with little effort, costs less than any other food per food value dollar, lasts several days without refrigeration, is low in calories, offers complete protein, and has been tested and used as both food and medicine for thousands of year.

Yet sprouts really are worth a million dollars in economic savings, health-giving qualities, variety, and great taste. With a jar, some water and a little effort, you can easily transform highly nutritious seeds, beans, and grains into delicious living vegetables loaded with vitamins, minerals, protein, enzymes, and natural fiber. Enzyme activity reaches its peak between the second and seventh day after sprouting. These young sprouts are the most nutritious.

Sprouted seeds, beans, grains and nuts are the only true "living foods." They are biogenic (life-generating). The life energy of living foods is liberated from the plant cells during the process of chewing and digestion, and becomes usable for the regeneration of your body.

A seed is the very core of life. It is a storehouse of concentrated energy and nutrients. Its food is held in reserve awaiting a suitable environment to begin growing. When conditions are met—proper temperature, oxygen and moisture—the miracle begins. An incredible flow of energy is released when a seed sprouts. Natural chemical changes occur. Starches in the seed are converted into simple sugars, proteins into simpler amino acids, fats into soluable fatty acids. Vitamins are created. In sprouting, all of the high-quality nutrients and enzymes in the seed, used to sustain the baby plant until it is able to draw nutrients from the soil, are made available to us in an easy-to-digest form.

SPROUTING IN HISTORY

The use of sprouted seeds for food and medicine is more than twice as old as the Great Wall of China. About 3000 B.C., the Emperor of China recorded their use in a book about medicinal herbs. Sprouted beans were prescribed for complaints such as edema, muscular cramps, visceral deficiencies, digestive disorders, weakness of the lungs, and problems involving the skin and hair. The Chinese and Japanese also sprouted mung, adzuki, soybeans, and barley as a part of their steady food supply.

In the West, sprouts were also used, first as medicine and later as food. Captain Cook's first completely successful extended ocean voyage lasted more than three years without losing a single man to the dreaded wasting disease called scurvy. Before Cook's famous voyage, most ships lost an average of half their crew to scurvy. Cook's secret was a specifically formulated low-heat malt made from sprouted beans. Today, sprouts are recognized as a specialty food, but during World War II the U.S. government was prepared to make soy sprouts an American staple. A campaign was launched to teach Americans how to sprout and prepare soybeans. The program began as a result of anticipated wartime shortages of protein, which never occurred. By 1948, soybeans and their sprouts were forgotten.

A few well-known scientists have published their findings on the value of sprouts as food and protective nutrition. Some of their conclusions are summarized below.

—Dr. C.Y. Tsai of Purdue University found that bean sprouts contain extraordinarily high levels of good-quality protein. Mung sprouts, for example, contain more than 25 percent of their calories as protein, which is a higher proportion than in T-bone steak. And soy sprouts have an even greater percentage. Because of their high levels of proteins (amino acids), vitamins, and minerals, Dr. Tsai considered sprouts to be one of the most perfect foods known to man.

—Dr. F. Grda of the University of Chicago demonstrated that a diet of sprouted beans, seeds, and grains, without recourse to other foods, was able to sustain life in animal experiments. Dr. Grda found that the vitamins, minerals, and proteins in sprouts are easily used by the body because they are supplied in a balanced and complete form. Moreover, Dr. Grda suggested that when sprouts are added to other foods, they make the nutrients in these foods more usable to the body as well.

—Dr. M. Beeskow of the Michigan Agricultural Experimental Station found an increased amount of Vitamin C in seeds after they were sprouted.

—Dr. C. Andrea of McGill University showed that sprouted peas contain 30 milligrams of Vitamin C per 100 grams (approximately 3½ ounces, a typical serving portion). Fresh-squeezed orange juice contains about 35 milligrams of Vitamin C per 100 grams.

—Dr. R. Bogert of the Kansas Agricultural Experimental Station measured 15 milligrams of Vitamin C in 40 grams of sprouted oats. That is more Vitamin C per weight than in fresh berries and honeydew melon.

—Dr. P.R. Burkholder of Yale University showed that when oats are sprouted, the Vitamin B_2 (riboflavin) content increases by 1300 percent, biotin by 50 percent, inositol by 50 percent, pantothenic acid by 200 percent, Vitamin B_6 (pyridoxine) by 500 percent, and folic acid by 600 percent. Because of these enormous increases over the vitamin content of dried grains and seeds, Dr. Burkholder recommended the wide-scale use of sprouts as food in the West.

—Dr. C. McCay of the Cornell University School of Nutrition was hired by the U.S. government during World War II to find suitable protein substitutes for meat, poultry, and dairy foods because of expected wartime shortages. After months of research, Dr. McCay concluded that sprouted soy and other beans would fill the need quite well. He wrote several articles that included instructions and recipes and were available through the U.S. Government Printing Office. Since the protein shortages never came, the campaign to educate Americans about the nutritional value of sprouts was dropped.

—Dr. F. Pottenger of the Price-Pottenger Nutrition Foundation was able to keep laboratory rats and guinea pigs alive through several generations on a diet of sprouted grains alone. Dr. Pottenger pronounced sprouted grains a complete food, able to support human life by themselves if the need arose. Other foods tested, such as cabbage, failed to sustain the animals after a number of weeks.

—Dr. C.F. Schnabel, a biochemist and independent agricultural consultant, found that sprouted wheat, by itself, was one of the only known foods that could sustain the life and health of experimental animals through generations. Dr. Schnabel was especially interested in sprouted wheat and wheatgrass as food for both farm animals and humans.

—Drs. C. Shaw and C.N. Lai of the University of Texas found that wheat, lentil, and mung sprouts were able to inhibit growth of cancer cells when a cancer-causing substance was exposed to healthy bacteria. According to the reseachers the key appears to be chlorophyll, which is found even more abundantly in greens and wheatgrass.

—Dr. J. Bland, professor of nutritional biochemistry at the University of Puget Sound, showed that approximately 6 cups (600 grams) of lentil sprouts supplied the recommended intake of protein for an adult male (50 grams). Dr. Bland concluded that sprouts could provide a significant portion of our daily protein needs in a safe and inexpensive form, compared to other plant and animal protein sources. In addition, he pointed out that as a bonus the person who eats sprouts on a regular basis also gets plenty of extra vitamins, enzymes, minerals and other vital nutrients.

Indeed, science has studied the potent sprouts as a prime food source and they have passed all the tests. Even more important, sprouts have proven their worth in human nutrition. For the thousands of people who have visited the Hippocrates Institute, and continue to rely on their nourishing properties, sprouts are a daily necessity—besides being fun to grow and care for.

GROWING SPROUTS

Almost any seed, grain, or legume can be sprouted for food, although some are tastier than others. Try all of the varieties listed in the chart at the end of this chapter. These include alfalfa, lentil, mung, soybean, and sunflower. Seeds can be purchased in natural food stores. Make sure that the seeds or grains have not been chemically treated, because if they have, the germination rate will drop. Broken or chipped seeds also will not sprout.

The basic care of sprouts involves keeping them moist and providing adequate drainage. Sprouts will mature more quickly in warm weather, so soaking times can be decreased and rinsing should be done more frequently to keep them cool. In colder weather, soak seeds longer and rinse them less frequently. The chart on pages 80–83 is based on a 70° F temperature. Since time and temperature determine when a seed reaches maturity, the times on the chart will vary as the temperature changes. Sprouts also respond to your energy. Given them love and they will love you by keeping your body healthy.

Equipment

You will need to buy very little equipment to begin your own sprout garden. If you opt for a modern automatic sprouter it can save you time and (eventually) money, and it will produce uniformly great sprouts every time. Nevertheless, manual sprouting can be taken care of in just minutes per week. You will need the following items:

Wide-mouth jars (such as Mason jars),
or sprout bags and bowls
Rubber bands

Mesh, plastic screening, or cheesecloth
cut in squares large enough to cover jar tops, or screened jar covers made especially for sprouting
Seeds or beans
Racks for draining jars

Instead of the bottle, mesh, and rubber hand you can purchase one of the many tray-type sprout growers, which consist of a plastic tray with small holes in the bottom (see illustration below).

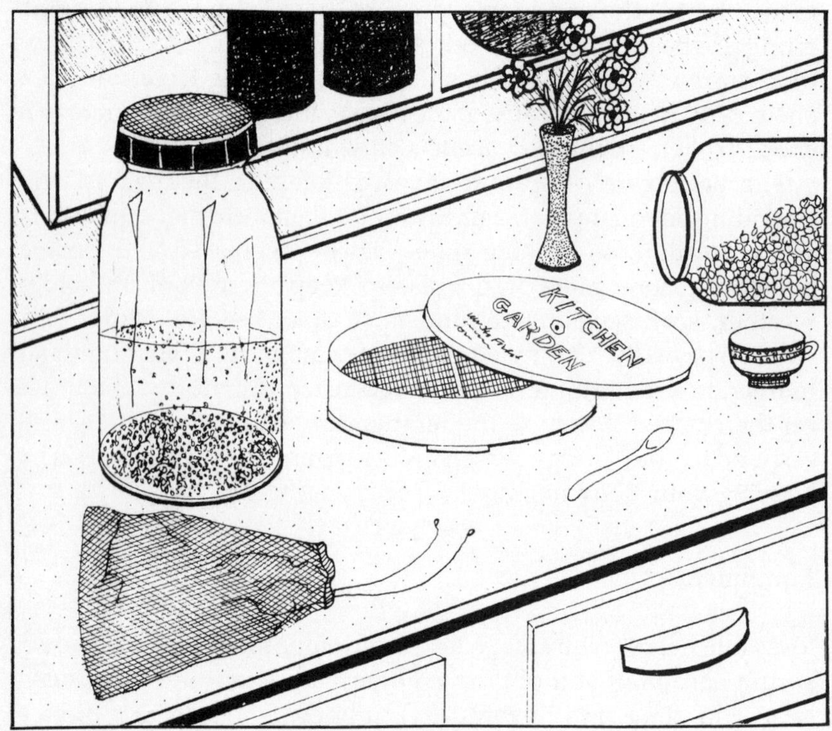

Tray-type sprouter.

Draining and Soaking

Put seeds in a jar and cover with a sprouting lid, mesh, or cheesecloth secured with a rubber band, or place seeds in a sprout bag and place in a bowl. To wash seeds, fill the container and then drain liquid. Then fill the jar or bowl about halfway with lukewarm water, preferably spring or filtered water.

Check the chart on pages 80–83 for recommended seed amounts and soaking times. Small seeds are soaked approximately four to six hours, larger seeds and beans eight to twelve hours. The larger the seed, the more time required. In general, small seeds should just cover the bottom of the jar. Bigger seeds should not fill the jar more than one-eighth full. Sprouts expand—for example, one pound of alfalfa seed produces eight pounds of sprouts.

After the seeds have been soaked, drain off the water. Fill the jar with fresh water. Foam will rise to the top. Sprouts should be rinsed until all this foam, which is caused by residue of the sprouting process, has been washed away.

Leave the jar upside down (45° angle) to ensure proper drainage and ventilation. Make sure that the opening isn't completely covered up by sprouts. If you are using a sprout bag, dip the whole bag in water several times and hang it up to drain.

If you are using a tray-type sprouter, place soaked seeds evenly in the bottom of the tray and cover it to keep out light. The sprouts will grow up evenly in carpet-like growth.

Rinsing

Rinse and drain sprouts well two or three times a day for three to five days. Use lukewarm water. Make sure that the sprouts are sufficiently drained, as too much water and too little air will lead to mold and spoilage. On the other hand, sprouts should never be allowed to dry out.

Very small seeds, such as alfalfa, may tend to mat up if packed too tightly. If this happens, they can be rinsed off in a basin of water. Hulls (the outside layer of seeds) will wash away at the same time.

When sprouting smaller seeds or mixes in a tray-type sprouter, remove the cover after three to four day's growth to allow light to reach the sprouts. When rinsing, make sure to rinse all the sprouts in the tray evenly and gently.

Harvesting

The best time to harvest sprouts is when they are at their peak, generally from one to five days (see Sprouting Chart, pp. 80–83). To harvest them, simply take sprouts from their tray or jar, and remove the hulls.

Lentils, hulled sunflowers, peas, and most grains do not need to be hulled. If you are using a tray-type sprouter, allow indirect light to reach the sprouts during the last two days of growth. As the leaves of the sprouts open, hulls will automatically be separated from the sprouts. Hulls of other seeds needn't be removed during the sprouting process, but they all should be washed off before use. Sprouts which are not hulled before storage tend to go bad.

To wash off hulls, place the sprouts in a sink and fill it with water. The hulls will rise to the surface and sprouts will sink to the bottom. Scoop the hulls from the surface and discard, reach underneath for the sprouts, and scoop them out of the water. Strain off the water and place the hulled sprouts in a jar. Rinsed sprouts can also be drained in sprouting bags.

Storage of Sprouts

Store hulled sprouts in refrigerator, in glass or plastic containers or bags. Always keep them covered. After harvesting, sprouts continue to grow in refrigerator at a very slow rate. If stored properly, they will last from seven to ten days.

The following sprout chart will be a handy reference when you are growing sprouts. It includes the essentials you will need to know to produce great sprouts, special growing tips, nutritional features of each variety, and suggested uses for your harvested sprouts.

A Note On Sprouting Mixology

Many of the members of the sprouting family are harmonious for growing in combination with others. When combining seeds for sprouting, follow these general rules for success. First, the seeds, beans or grains used must have a similar rate of growth. Second, use the flavor of the original seeds to determine the percentages of each used in the mixes. You can mix grains such as wheat, rye, and triticale; medium-sized seeds and beans such as lentil, adzuki, and chick pea; or smaller seeds such as alfalfa, cabbage, and clover. Create your own combinations to suit your own tastes and nutritional needs. Use the same sprouting methods for combinations as for single seeds.

Sprouting Mixology

Variety	Soak (hours)	Dry Measure	Length at Harvest	Ready in (days)	Sprouting Tips
Adzuki	12	1 cup	½–1″	3–5	Easy sprouter. Try short & long.
Alfalfa	4–6	3 table-spoons	1–1½″	4–5	Place in light to develop chlorophyll 1–2 days before harvest.
Almond	12	1 cup	0″	1	Swells up, does not sprout.
Cabbage	4–6	⅓ cup	1″	4–5	Develops chlorophyll when mature.
Chick Pea	12	1 cup	½″	2–3	Mix with lentils & wheat, or use alone.
Clover	4–6	3 table-spoons	1–1½″	4–5	Mix with other seeds. Develops chlorophyll.
Corn	12	1 cup	½″	2–3	Use sweet corn. Try short & long.
Fenugreek	8	½ cup	½–1″	3–5	Pungent flavor; mix with other seeds.
Green Pea	12	1 cup	½″	2–3	Use whole peas.
Lentil	12	½ cup	¼–¾″	3–5	Earthy flavor. Try short & long. Versatile sprout.
Millet	8	1 cup	¼″	2–3	Use unhulled type.
Mung	12	½ cup	½–1½″	3–5	Grow in dark. When rinsing, soak in cold water for 1 minute.

Nutritional Highlights	Suggested Uses
rich in protein, iron, & calcium	salads, Oriental dishes, loaves, sandwiches, casseroles
complete protein, vitamins A, B, C, D, E, F, K, rich in minerals	salads, sandwiches, juices, soups, dressings
rich in protein, calcium, and fats	salads, cereals, soups, breads, dressings, sauces, desserts
rich in minerals and vitamins A & C	cole slaw, salads, sandwiches, soups
complete protein, minerals	dips, spreads, casseroles, salads, loaves, breads
protein, vitamins, and minerals	salads, sandwiches, breads, soups
protein, vitamins B & E, fiber, minerals	breads, granola, snacks, cereals, grain dishes
rich in iron, vitamin A, & protein	soups, curries, salads, loaves, casseroles
rich in protein, minerals, vitamins B & C	dips, soups, loaves, casseroles, salads
complete protein, minerals, B vitamins	salads, soups, breads, loaves, spreads, casseroles, curries
vitamins A & B, protein, fiber	breads, cereals, soups, salads, casseroles
complete protein, vitamins A, B, & C, minerals	Oriental dishes, soups, juices, sandwiches, salads, loaves

Variety	Soak (hours)	Dry Measure	Length at Harvest	Ready in (days)	Sprouting Tips
Mustard	4–6	¼ cup	1″	4–5	Hot flavor; mix with other seeds.
Oats	12	1 cup	¼–½″	2–3	Find whole sprouting type.
Radish	4–6	¼ cup	1″	4–5	Hot flavor; mix with other seeds. Develops chlorophyll.
Rye	12	1 cup	¼–½″	2–3	Try mixing with wheat & lentils.
Sesame	4–6	1 cup	0″	1–2	Tiny sprout, turns bitter if left too long.
Soybean	12	½ cup	½″	2	Rinse often. Try short & long.
Sunflower	8	2 cups	0–½″	1–3	Use hulled seeds. Mix with alfalfa & grow 4–5 days.
Triticale	12	1 cup	¼–½″	2–3	A grain hybrid like wheat.
Watercress	4–6	4 tablespoons	½″	4–5	Spicy; mix with other seeds.
Wheat	12	1 cup	¼–½″	2–3	Try short & long. For sweeter taste, mix with other seeds.

Nutritional Highlights	Suggested Uses
mustard oil, vitamins, minerals	salads, sandwiches, juices, soups
protein, vitamin A, alkaline minerals, fiber	breads, cereals, soups, loaves, casseroles, grain dishes
potassium, vitamin C	salads, sandwiches, Mexican-style food, soups, dressings
vitamins B & E, minerals, protein	cereals, breads, salads, milks, soups, granola
rich in protein, calcium, vitamins A & E, fats, fiber	dressings, milks, salads, breads, cereals, desserts
complete protein, minerals, vitamins A, B, C, & E, lecithin	soups, casseroles, breads, salads, milks, Oriental dishes
rich in minerals, fats, protein, vitamins B, D, & E	dressings, salads, soups, breads, cereals, desserts, milks
see wheat	*see* wheat
vitamins, minerals	salads, sandwiches, breads, garnishes
vitamins B, C, & E, minerals, complete protein	salads, cereals, soups, milks, breads, desserts, granola, snacks

8

Wheatgrass Miracles

I can imagine waking up and reading this story in the morning newspaper:

> **Fountain of Youth Discovered by Team of Explorers**
>
> Deep in the jungles of Kahoulawassi, Banga, a group of researchers led by Emil Hogarth discovered what may turn out to be the fountain of youth. The group set out a month ago to investigate the legendary Kobobo tribe. The youngest Kobobo were reported to live at least 150 years. Four day's journey into the jungle the researchers spotted their first Kobobo, a surprisingly agile older man who, upon seeing the foreigners, sprang away into the jungle.
>
> Two more days passed before John Reynolds, a member of the expedition, literally stumbled upon what may be the Kobobo's secret of youth. Tracking footprints, Reynolds fell into a pool of dark green liquid. He noticed an oddly shaped device resembling an old-fashioned well pump with ten or more clay pitchers under its spout. Green-stained and dripping wet, he moved the handle of the pump a few times, until more of the green elixir issued forth.
>
> When they heard of the discovery, the team decided to hide and wait for the Kobobo to return. Early the next morning, two well-built Kobobo men arrived at the green hole. They filled several of the clay pitchers with the green liquid and carried them away on a stick placed between their shoulders. . . .

Laboratory analysis of the green fluid, which the team observed the Kobobo drinking five times a day, revealed it to be a chlorophyll protein derived from algae, similar to the liquid chlorophyll extracted from ordinary green leaves or grasses. It had a sweet taste but was too strong for the explorers to consume in quantity, although they drank as much as they could.

Upon reaching the mainland, the team was examined routinely for jungle parasites and infection. Much to the surprise of the examining physician, two members of the team had normalized their blood pressure. Another had healed completely of a nasty leg sore, and a fourth had cured himself of a bothersome stomach ulcer. All of the men had little appetite for food and reportedly felt terrific despite the 200-mile trek without modern conveniences. The physician concluded that exercise and adventure were responsible for their miracle cures.

According to Hogarth, however, all the team could think about was the pool of sweet green liquid that they had discovered in the jungle.

Of course, this is not a true story, but it has an intuitive appeal. Think of how much energy and power you would have if you could harness the nutritious chlorophyll in green grass and herbs. Instinctively, all humans seek green. When spring arrives, we feel refreshed to see the landscape covered with green, and are refreshed by the crispness of the oxygen-rich air. Were it not for the green of spring and summer, animals or humans could not exist. Even in the deserts of the world, underground water supplies give life to greenery, which in turn provides creatures with water, protection and nourishment. Areas where no trees or grasses are found could truly be considered wastelands.

Inner-city ghettos are virtually man-created wastelands. Few trees, plants, and birds and hardly any wildlife survives there. Even the light of day scarcely creeps through the buildings in some places. The highest rates of crime, disease, schizophrenia, drug abuse, alcoholism, pollution, and suicide also characterize this unwholesome and unsettling environment.

It's no wonder city people crave the country or the suburbs. Green fields and tree-covered mountains have a calming, regenerating effect on our nervous system and thinking. Intuitively, we seek our biological "roots"—green leaves and grasses—for rest from the often maddening pace of modern life.

Trees, grasses, and all growing plants absorb water, minerals, and gasses from the soil and air and convert these, through the process known as photosynthesis, into carbohydrates, proteins, and energy. These are stored in the plants. No other living thing has this ability to capture the sun's energy and utilize soil nutrients to synthesize matter and energy. Plants also absorb carbon dioxide gasses, which can be poisonous to humans, and excrete oxygen. (Humans, on the other hand, breathe oxygen and exhale carbon dioxide.) Without green plants, there would be no oxygen and no living things on Earth.

GRASSES: FOOD AND MEDICINE

More than fifty million years ago, grasses spread over the Earth and created a major reorganization of the animal world. Those animals that could take advantage of its nourishing qualities thrived. From the chlorophyll the grasses contained, they were able to build blood, flesh, and bones; they became the most powerful animals on Earth. In the present day, elephants, moose, horses, elk, oxen, bulls, and others grow strong and sustain their huge bodies by eating grasses and other herbs. And although humans do not have the ability to break down and digest large quantities of grass fibers, many medical researchers believe chlorophyll extracts (juice) to be an excellent natural treatment for a number of diverse ailments.

The medicinal use of grasses is thousands of years old. In the Orient, grasses and the chlorophyll extracted from them were used for many complaints. Since biblical days, grasses and preparations made from them have been used by Western nature healers, herbalists, physicians (until recently), and native local healers. In the nineteenth century, it wouldn't have been a surprise if grandma wrapped a crushed grass poultice around a broken or injured leg.

In the early part of this century, chlorophyll was regarded as a top-notch weapon in the arsenal of pharmocopia. Many physicians used it in the treatment of various complaints such as ulcers and skin disease, and as a pain reliever and breath freshener. One report by Dr. Benjamine Gurskin, then director of experimental pathology at Temple University, was published in the *American Journal of Surgery*. Dr. Gurskin discussed more than 1000 cases in which various disorders were treated with chlorophyll. Commenting on his associates' experience with chlorophyll, he wrote, "It is interesting to note that there is not a single case recorded in which either improvement or cure has not taken place." In 1949, *Reader's Digest* published an article called "The Mysterious Power of Chlorophyll," which discussed the tremendous potential of chlorophyll as a food and medicine.

After World War II, however, chlorophyll and many other natural antiseptics were replaced by the faster-acting antibiotics and chemical antiseptics. The few preparations that remained for sale were limited to breath fresheners and "health" supplements. Today, chlorophyll from grasses is receiving a great deal of renewed interest, especially among health circles. Seven-inch-tall wheatgrass (and its juice) has several definite missions to perform in the bodies of modern men: blood alkalization, cleansing, and generation and oxygenation of red blood cells. It may also have a number of vital healing functions. And when it is used properly, there are no side effects.

CHLOROPHYLL AND OXYGEN

One of chlorophyll's more important functions in the Hippocrates Diet is oxygenation of the bloodstream. On a high-fat and high-protein diet our oxygen supply is reduced. Dr. John Gainer, reporting in *Science News*, August, 1971, stated that even a moderate increase in blood plasma protein can reduce oxygen levels of the blood by as much as 60 percent. I have found that without sufficient oxygen in our blood we develop symptoms of low energy, sluggish digestion, and metabolism. In essence, we are unable to oxidize or burn up food efficiently. Unable to digest, assimilate and eliminate thoroughly its old fuel, with a weakened immune system and reduced blood oxygen level, the body becomes ripe for cancer. In his book, *The Cause And Prevention Of Cancer*, Dr. Otto Warburg, winner of a Nobel prize for physiology and medicine (1931) concluded that oxygen deprivation was a major cause of cancer and that with a steady blood supply of oxygen to all the cells, cancer could be prevented indefinitely.

There are many ways to bring increased oxygen into the blood, but without first eliminating the causes of oxygen deprivation (such as smoking, high-fat and high-protein cooked foods, alcohol, drugs, poor breathing, and sedentary habits), any attempt to oxygenate the blood will fail. And we must bring renewed oxygen into the blood to effect a significant degree of physical regeneration.

Breathing exercises, walking, and diet are the safest ways to oxygenate the blood. Exercises with controlled breathing increase our vital lung capacity, bringing more oxygen into the bloodstream. Walking helps to increase circulation of oxygen to all parts of the body. As for diet, all fresh raw vegetables, fruits, sprouts, and greens, especially wheatgrass, have oxygen contained in liquid. When we eat, or juice and drink these foods, our blood supply of oxygen increases. Dr. Norman Walker, a centenarian health researcher, has been living primarily on fruits and vegetables for over sixty years. He feels his longevity is due in large part of the liquid oxygen, enzymes and chlorophyll contained in fresh juices.

Chlorophyll is the "blood" of the plant. It is the protein in plant life that gives it its distinctive green or purple color. When compared to a molecule of hemoglobin, the oxygen carrier in human blood, chlorophyll is almost identical. The major difference, as you can see below, is that the nucleus of chlorophyll contains magnesium (Mg), whereas hemoglobin contains iron (Fe).

Of course, I am not attempting to lead you to the conclusion that you should live exclusively on green leaves, herbs and grasses, and become as strong or as big as an elephant. But, by taking a percentage of green foods and juices each day, especially wheatgrass, you can add vital nutrients such as minerals, enzymes, vitamins, oxygen, and protein to your blood. Healthier blood can lead only to a healthier, more vital body, better able to withstand stress without injury. Let's take a brief look at what scientists have to say about chlorophyll and wheatgrass juice.

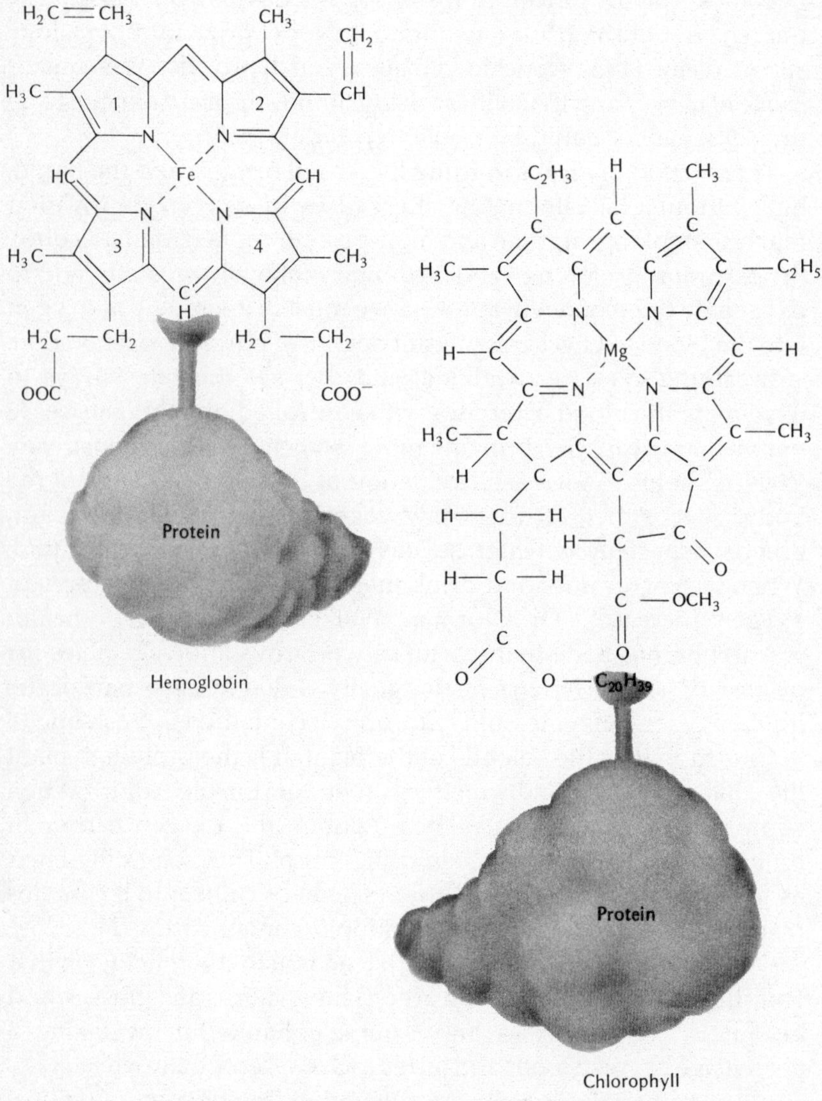

Hemoglobin

Chlorophyll

A Comparison of Chlorophyll Molecule and Hemoglobin.

From *Biology: A Human Approach*, by Irwin W. and Vilia G. Sherman. Copyright© 1975 by Oxford University Press, Inc. Reproduced by permission.

CHLOROPHYLL AND GRASSES IN RESEARCH

Many of the experimental studies of chlorophyll were performed before the 1950s. At that time the use of chlorophyll in medicine had reached its peak. Unfortunately, liquid chlorophyll turned out to be highly unstable; it could not be bottled and stored for more than a few hours, making it impractical as a pharmaceutical. A synthetic chlorophyll extract which was produced by fermenting fresh chlorophyll and bonding it with certain mineral elements proved to be inconsistent and at times productive of side effects. Chlorophyll as a treatment was then for the most part abandoned by the medical profession, despite the dramatic effects indicated in the various studies that are summarized below.

—J.H. Hughs and A.L. Latner, University of Liverpool scientists reporting in the *Journal of Physiology*, performed several experiments using rabbits. In their study, rabbits were made anemic by daily bleeding and were given various doses of boiled (refined) and unrefined fresh chlorophyll. The results showed the rabbits' ability to convert chlorophyll into hemoglobin, correcting the anemia, especially where the fresh chlorophyll was used.

—Drs. R. Redpath and T.C. Davis, eye, ear, nose and throat specialists at Temple University, treated and cured over one thousand cases of sinusitis, head colds, rhinitis, respiratory infections, etc., with chlorophyll. Their results were discussed in an article published in the *Science Newsletter*, 1941.

—Drs. H.A. Rafsky and C.I. Krieger, reported a case study in the *Review of Gastroenterology*, 1948, in which twenty people with colon disorders, several of whom suffered from ulcerative colitis, were given chlorophyll implants for treatment. Definite improvement was seen in a majority of the cases.

—Drs. L.W. Smith and A.E. Livingston, in the 1943 *American Journal of Surgery*, reported a study in which 1372 animals were wounded surgically. The application of chlorophyll to the wounds of some of these animals sped the rate of healing and recovery by 25 percent over the control (untreated) group. The ability to inhibit detrimental bacterial growth on the wounds was also clearly demonstrated.

—M. Lourou and O. Lartigue published a paper in *Experientia,* 1950, showing that green cabbage, when added to the ordinary chow diet of guinea pigs, increased their resistance to lethal X-rays. The usual signs of radiation poisoning were prevented or delayed in the pigs eating the cabbage as a dietary supplement.

—H. Spector and D.H. Colloway, researching the effects of radiation on guinea pigs for the U.S. Army, repeated Lourou and Lartigues' experiment using broccoli and alfalfa and got the same results—the effects of lethal doses of radiation were slowed when greens were added to the chow diet.

—Dr. E. Krebs, discoverer of Vitamin B_{17} or laetrile, found that the Vitamin B_{17} content of seeds increased up to 100 times when they sprouted. Krebs has identified almonds, sprouts, and wheatgrass as good sources of Vitamin B_{17}. Vitamin B_{17} aids in growth and development, assists the nervous system, and may inhibit the proliferation of cancer cells.

—Dr. G.H. Earp Thomas, a biochemist at Bloomfield Laboratories, after researching the nutritional properties of wheatgrass juice, stated in a letter to me that it was perhaps "the richest nutritional liquid known to man."

—P. Altman and D. Dittmer, writing in *Metabolism,* summarized separate studies by Sprague, Crampton, and Harris, reporting that wheatgrass is an excellent source of calcium, chlorine, iron, magnesium, potassium, phosphorous, sulfur, cobalt, and zinc, making it a highly alkalizing substance capable of reducing the excess acid in the blood of modern people.

—Dr. Y. Hagiwara found dried barley grass juice to contain 60 times more Vitamin C than oranges and 8 times more iron than spinach. He has used chlorophyll extract to alleviate symptoms in patients with hypertension, obesity, atopic dermatitis, pancreatitis, and peptic ulcer.

From the medical evidence, and years of experience in observing people with all kinds of problems alleviate their symptoms using fresh chlorophyll from wheatgrass, I am convinced that young grasses, alfalfa, and other chlorophyll-rich plants are a safe and effective alternative treatment for ailments such as high blood pressure, obesity, diabetes, gastritis, ulcers, pancreas and liver problems, osteomyelitis, asthma, eczema, hemorrhoids, skin problems, fatigue, anemia, halitosis, body odor, and constipation. I have found chlorophyll to be effective in alleviating symptoms of oral infection, bleeding gums, burns, athlete's foot, and cancer. Moreover, used as a nutritional supplement, it has also shown a tremendous ability to prevent a number of problems. And it is no mystery why.

WHEATGRASS: A PRIME SOURCE OF CHLOROPHYLL

The following data on the nutrients contained by first joint wheatgrass (7–10″ tall) is taken from a report Dr. C.F. Schnabel made to the American Chemical Society.

	Nutrient	Milligrams per pound (453.59 g)
	Chlorophyll	5000 mg
	Choline	4000
	Vitamin C (ascorbic acid)	2000
	Vitamin A (carotene)	360
	Vitamin E	120
	Vitamin F	120
	Vitamin K	120
	Niacin	120
B vitamins	Vitamin B_2 (riboflavin)	24
B vitamins	Vitamin B_1 (thiamine)	12
B vitamins	Pantothenic acid	8
B vitamins	Vitamin B_6	4

It may seem that wheatgrass contains relatively small amounts of the B vitamins, but in actuality the amounts compare favorably with the latest research on Vitamin B needs as compared to C and A. All in all, wheatgrass juice is a potent food/medicine that has many uses.

JUICING WHEATGRASS

Since wheatgrass is so fibrous, and its fiber is indigestible by humans, we always use it juiced. You could use your teeth to juice the grass by chewing it and spitting out the pulp, but to get several ounces by this method would wear out your jaw, and your patience! It is far better to purchase a slow-turning juicer made especially for juicing sprouts, greens, soft vegetables and wheatgrass. Both hand-crank and electric units are available. I recommend the electric model, as to get several ounces of juice by hand is tiring and takes a lot longer. Besides, the hand units tend to wind up collecting dust on the closet shelf much more often than the electric models do.

Buckwheat and sunflower greens can be juiced in the same way, along with sprouts and vegetables to make what I call "green drinks," or they can be added to salads and other live food recipes.

With your electric juicer on, merely place a bunch of cut grass, about three-quarters of an inch in diameter, tip down into the hole at the top. The juicer will do the rest. A few drops of juice will come out of the front of the juicer, followed by the pulp. The juice itself will come out the spout on the bottom of the machine. I like to run the pulp through the juicer two or more times to get as much juice as possible from it. After each use, be sure to take your juicer apart and wash and dry all the parts with a non-detergent soap.

If you can't afford an electric wheatgrass juicer, but you still want to use wheatgrass juice, you can try running it through a meat grinder (which costs about as much as a hand juicer) and squeeze the mashed pulp through a piece of cheesecloth to extract the juice. However, if you are committed to using wheatgrass and green drinks on a regular basis, an electric wheatgrass juicer is essential equipment.

Wheatgrass juice is very volatile. It should be used within twelve hours.

USES OF WHEATGRASS CHLOROPHYLL

Like all foods, wheatgrass, greens and other grasses lose much of their potency when processed. We recommend, therefore, the use of freshly squeezed or pressed chlorophyll preparations over dried, powdered or bottled types. It is also best to obtain organically grown greens or wheatgrass for juicing. I have found wheatgrass to be fastest-growing and most nutritious grass. Wheatgrass juice has unlimited applications. There are basically two ways to use it, however, internally (orally), and externally.

Internal use of wheatgrass chlorophyll helps to cleanse the blood, organs, and gastrointestinal tract of debris. It stimulates metabolism and bodily enzyme systems in enriching the blood by increasing red blood cell count, and in dilating the blood pathways throughout the body, reducing blood pressure. Wheatgrass aids the glands—especially the pituitary and pancreas—in normalizing their functions, and that is important in combating obesity and indigestion.

As a protective food/medicine, wheatgrass chlorophyll is a powerhouse of vitamins, minerals, amino acids and oxygen—a great nutritional supplement. But it doesn't stop there. Wheatgrass chlorophyll aids digestion and can also be used to relieve many internal pains. It has been used to treat peptic ulcer and ulcerative colitis. Another important use is protective alkalization of the blood. Reducing conditions of overacidity, the alkaline-forming properties of wheatgrass juice help to strengthen the blood and body against invading germs. When implanted rectally, wheatgrass chlorophyll helps to cleanse and stimulate the colon, restoring minerals and strengthening its muscular walls.

There are several ways wheatgrass juice may be used externally. For first aid, you should always have access to some wheatgrass so that you can squeeze juice for applying to burns, cuts, rashes, poison ivy, and insect bites. The juice can be soaked up in a lump of semi-dried grass and placed in a bandage to help heal boils, open sores, external ulcers, tumors, and other skin problems. The poultice will have a soothing, drawing effect. Applied to the skin and scalp, wheatgrass juice acts as a disinfectant, a skin food (a portion of it is absorbed into the blood), and tightener for loose, sagging skin. On the hair, it can be used either before or after shampooing. Try leaving it on for a couple of hours—it will help to mend damaged hair and correct itchy or scaly scalp problems.

Wheatgrass juice can be chewed or gargled to freshen stale breath or relieve sore throats. If chewed and applied to a sore tooth or to the gums, it will help reduce swelling and pain. Rubbed into the gums, it can help remedy pyorrhea and bleeding.

An effective eye wash for the relief of eyestrain and itchiness can be made from finely strained wheatgrass juice. Apply the juice with a dropper or purchase an eyecup at a drugstore. When placed in the ear with a dropper, strained wheatgrass juice helps reduce the pressure and discomfort of many an earache. If drops are inserted into the sinuses and inhaled, it will help cleanse and open nasal passages. When using wheatgrass juice in these sensitive areas, you may experience a temporary worsening of symptoms. Your eyes may be even more itchy and red or your sinuses may clog further, but be assured that these reactions are temporary and will improve greatly a few minutes later. At the Institute, we regard such reactions as a positive sign—that is, as an indication that the body is being cleansed of unwholesome substances. However, you may try using less wheatgrass juice next time, and diluting it with some water. Also try using wheatgrass in the many other ways it can be used outside the body. If reactions persist, discontinue use.

As a sleep aid, merely place a tray of living wheatgrass near the head of your bed. It will enhance the oxygen in the air and generate healthful negative ions to help you sleep more soundly. I have seen remarkable results when insomniacs have placed just one or two trays of wheatgrass by their beds.

Over the years, many of my pets—dogs, cats, birds, monkeys, and gerbils have also benefited from wheatgrass. Both when ill and when healthy, these animals would eat the wheatgrass directly off the tray or eat grass I placed in their food. Along with sprouts chopped into their food, wheatgrass will help keep pets healthy and happy.

In laboratory experiments performed by the late G.H. Earp Thomas of Bloomfield Labs in New Jersey, wheatgrass juice was able to neutralize sodium fluoride, a compound that is added to the municipal drinking water in many communities. Fluoridation was originally introduced as a means of preventing tooth decay, but there is evidence that it does more harm than good. Another widespread use of sodium fluoride is as a rat and roach poison. Wheatgrass juice is by no means a replacement for the proper home refiltering of city water, a procedure that we recommend at the Hippocrates Institute. But it can improve the quality of the tap water used to grow houseplants, sprouts, wheatgrass, and greens, or to feed pets. Spring or filtered water is preferred for drinking and addition directly to our food supply. Furthermore, although no hard data has been compiled, hair mineral analyses of guests at the Hippocrates Institute indicate that wheatgrass juice has the ability to draw toxic metals from the blood and tissues.

DOSAGES

In terms of dosages, a word of caution is appropriate before ending this chapter. Many times enthusiastic students will drink eight or more ounces of wheatgrass juice—in one sitting—their first day at the Institute. In most cases, they will feel sick and have to lie down for a while. Some of them have even vomited, vowing not to use the juice again, ever. Of course, that is the wrong way to approach wheatgrass juice. If it is to be used, one to two ounces should be sipped slowly, either straight or mixed with other juices or water. On the healing regime, the one to two ounces can be taken three to four times per day—always on an empty or nearly empty stomach. Smaller doses, frequently swished around the mouth with the saliva, will attune the body to the juice and will not cause stomach upset.

A food or herb used every day week after week will lose effectiveness as a medicine unless periodic breaks from use are taken, allowing the body's adaptive mechanisms to relax themselves. Even when you are on the building/maintenance program, discontinue the oral use of wheatgrass juice for a couple of days per week and for an entire week per month to allow the body to readjust.

In external use, fresh juice or fresh poultices should be placed every two to four hours on the affected body part. A bandage with a towel and plastic wrapped around the poultice will hold it on the body and keep it moist. Clean the area periodically with castile soap and let it breathe a few minutes before reapplication. Again, periodically give the area a break from use if treatment lasts longer than a couple of weeks.

If I have made it seem like wheatgrass juice is a panacea, it is not. It is no replacement for a healthy lifestyle, high-quality living food, and the other Hippocrates principles I have outlined. Used as a cure-all along with combinations of bad-quality and toxic foods, it will do little to help. It is merely a powerful tool that can be aimed against the enemy, overpowering it without drastic side effects. Wheatgrass juice works best along with the important health guidelines we have already discussed, and with food combining our next topic of discussion.

9

Apples And Oranges Aren't The Same

For many years it was believed by scientists and lay people alike that the stomach could not tell one food from another, and that it digested one combination of foods as well as it did any other. Today we know that this is wrong, and yet, the majority of people still acts as if it's true. Most of us eat combinations of foods that cause digestive distress, and then reach for a dose of alkalizers to quiet our upset stomachs. The fact that antacids are the largest-selling over-the-counter drug is evidence that something is wrong with the way we eat.

Yet, while we do know that proper food combining is important for good health, the simple rules I will share with you probably wouldn't be much help to the average eater because his diet is so poor. You and I might agree that meats, ice cream, cake, coffee or tea, fried potatoes, and canned vegetables shouldn't be eaten in the same meal, for these things need not be eaten at all. The danger in eating two, three, or more of them lies in the fact that each one of them is toxic and unnatural.

On the other hand, what harm could there be in eating a salad of cabbage, lettuce, sprouts, carrots, cucumber and sprouted nuts? Let's review briefly what happens to food that enters the body.

DIGESTION

The human gastrointestinal tract is about thirty feet long. The processes of digestion, assimilation, and elimination take place in different stages along the gastrointestinal tract. Our food must go through special predigestive stages before it can be assimilated and used as fuel. Carbohydrates (starches) become simple sugars, fats become fatty acids, and proteins break down into amino acids. The entire process of digestion culminating in elimination takes sixteen to twenty-four hours in a healthy adult (as compared with an average thirty-six to seventy-two hours for the average American).

The more food is chewed, the more active are the salivary glands located in and around the mouth. Their function is to secrete enzymes which aid in the predigestion of starches. But they can only do their job when food is well chewed (masticated), so proper chewing is very important.

Once masticated, the food enters the first chamber of the stomach where it will sit for up to one hour while food and salivary enzymes continue to predigest it. Slowly the food descends into the tide of acid digestive juices produced deeper in the stomach, where it is churned from side to side and saturated with the juices.

Some food particles and liquids are absorbed directly through the stomach wall. Ninety percent of the food, however, remains in the stomach undergoing protein digestion before moving into the small intestine.

The small intestine is accordian-like for maximum surface area. Millions of finger-like tentacles called villi line its interior walls. Their job is to absorb nutrients. Once absorbed, the nutrients are transported to the liver where they are filtered into the bloodstream and transformed into elements needed by the body. From the liver the food (now blood) is sent to the lungs, where it picks up a fresh supply of oxygen before being sent out to every cell of the body. Can you imagine having to make such a journey each day just to get to work?

In the meantime, undigested food residues and fiber move into the colon for the absorption of available minerals and liquids. After this final stage of digestion, wastes are eliminated from the body.

FOOD COMBINATIONS

A detailed look at digestive physiology reveals the fact that different foods are acted upon differently by the digestive system.

Starchy foods, for example, require alkaline digestive juices which are supplied initially in the mouth. Protein foods require the acidic juices formed in the stomach. When the acids mix with the alkaline juices they tend to neutralize each other. Thus, the mixing of starches and protein foods at the same meal slows digestion of both and indigestion occurs.

To avoid any form of indigestion and to ensure optimal assimilation on the Hippocrates Diet, it is important to follow these simple rules for combining foods (see the chart on page 103 for specific examples):

- Fruits and vegetables don't mix. The sugars and acids in fruits slow the digestion of the starches in vegetables and may cause fermentation, bloating and gas. It is best to eat fruits and vegetables separately at different meals. Occasional fruit desserts should be eaten 1½–2 hours after a meal of vegetables or sprouts.
- When eating fruits, avoid mixing acid fruits with sweet fruits. Use either sweet *or* acid fruits with subacid fruits.
- Any greens, sprouts, and vegetables (including avocados) mix well together. Sauces made from avocados, seeds, or nuts also mix well with greens, vegetables, and sprouts. Just try to avoid using overly complex mixtures of these foods at one meal. A good rule of thumb is to limit the number of foods used in combination to 8 or less.
- Avoid eating breads, sprouted grains or grain crisps with acid fruits. Occasionally you may use sweet or subacid fruits with sprouted grains to make cereals or breads.
- Fruits go well with sprouted seed or nut sauces. The one exception is melons, which should be eaten only with other melons or alone.
- Try to avoid drinking with your meals. It is better to take juices ½ hour before meals or 1½ hours after. Drinking while eating weakens the action of the digestive juices in the stomach and is unnecessary in terms of thirst when you eat plenty of natural foods, because they have a high percentage of water.

For optimal digestion, also try to:

- Chew your food thoroughly, 30 or more chews per mouthful. Mix liquids and juices with your saliva as well.
- Eat food that is warmed to room temperature. Excessively cold foods dilate the diaphragm, which can cause chest pains. Another reason to avoid cold food is that it must be brought to body temperature before it can be digested, and it requires an expenditure of your own body heat to warm it.
- Eat raw food at a meal before any cooked food. Otherwise the cooked food eaten holds up the digestion of the raw and the latter can ferment, causing uncomfortable gas.
- Be as relaxed as possible when eating, and when you can, for a time afterwards as well.

The chart that follows summarizes the most important rules of combining foods in the Hippocrates Diet. While I have found this simple advice helpful and correct for myself and others, it is important to tune into your own needs, likes and dislikes as you see fit. As long as the foods you eat each day conform to the overall dietary guidelines outlined in Chapter 1 you can be assured of getting all of the required nutrients (see Appendix) in your diet.

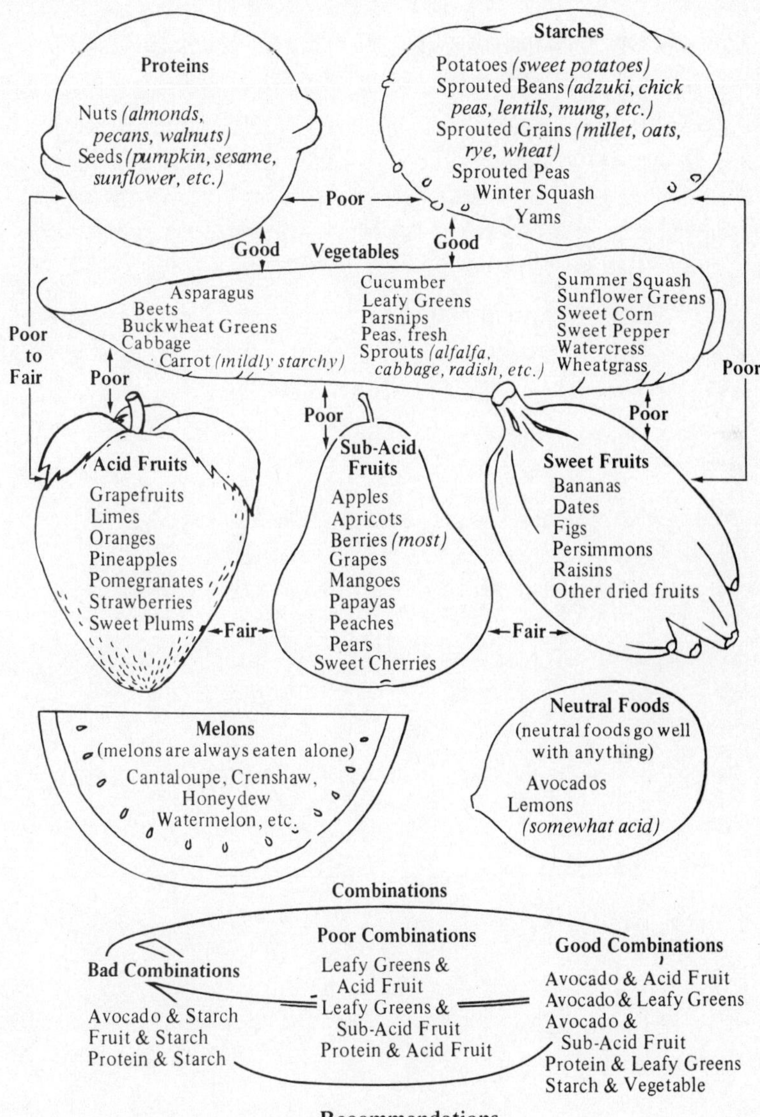

Recommendations

- Make meals of one or two combinations, especially one protein or starch with one or two vegetables.
- All juices can be mixed because they are liquid and will be absorbed by the body in ½ hour.

Food Combining Chart

10

Hippocrates Diet Recipes

THE HIPPOCRATES KITCHEN

Preparing nutritionally balanced and tasty food is a challenge no matter what your diet is. A few important guidelines about kitchen setup, equipment and how to use it, and basic foods to have on hand for the Hippocrates Diet will save you lots of time and energy, and may mean the difference between mediocre and fantastic results.

You will need to make an investment in a few kitchen appliances. If you have them already, great; if not, don't worry—they will pay for themselves in more ways than you can imagine. A good quality multi-speed blender will frequently be used for making dressings, sauces, cheeses, yogurts, soups, and so on, as will a good vegetable juicer. Keep in mind that a blender cannot substitute for a juicer, as a blender merely liquefies the fruit or vegetable, while the juicer removes the juices and separates them from the pulp. I recommend a Champion Juicer because of its many uses, such as extracting fruit and vegetable juices, making nut butters, vegetable loaves and spreads, bread dough, dried fruit candies, seed milks, and, most importantly, fruit ice cream. The Norwalk Juicer and the Acme Juicer are other models that are also used at the Institute.

Because of the highly fibrous nature of many grasses, greens, and sprouts, you will need to have a slow-turning juicer to juice them. This is different from the high-speed juicers mentioned above. For more information about the slow-turning wheatgrass juicers made especially for the Hippocrates Institute, write to us for details. Hand, electric, and convertible models are available. If you are serious about following the Hippocrates Diet, you will need two kinds of juicers, (slow and fast turning), and a blender.

For making sauerkraut and other fermented vegetable dishes, you will need a crock or large bowl, a plate that fits inside it, a brick or other weight, a baseball bat or sanded 2″ × 4″ board, and a bucket to pound the cabbage in. To powder herbs for this and other recipes, it is also helpful to have a hard spice grinder or electric coffee mill. The coffee mill can double as a seed and nut mill and is inexpensive and handy to have around. You will also need a couple of sharp vegetable knives, a good-sized cutting board, and a vegetable grater to make salads. A stainless-steel strainer is indispensable, and a bamboo sushi roller is also recommended.

The planting supplies listed in Chapter 6 (trays, oil, and seeds) and the sprouting supplies listed in Chapter 7 (jars and seeds), are also essential. If you absolutely cannot foresee planting greens and wheatgrass for lack of space or other reasons, try to find someone in your area who grows and sells greens and wheatgrass.

The last piece of equipment you will need is a dehydrator. This can replace your oven and is useful for drying vegetable chips, breads and grain crisps, fruits (when they are cheap and in season), pie crusts, and seed loaves.

After you get the feel of the recipes and preparation techniques, you will be spending only half the time you now spend in the kitchen. And if you love working in the kitchen—like I do—and make lots of especially creative dishes, you will do more with less time. By not having to cook meals and wash greasy dishes, you will conserve time that you can use to shop for high-quality food, tend sprouts and greens, and relax and/or exercise.

If you are concerned about where you are going to put all the extra equipment, don't worry—I've stored some of mine in the oven! You may have to keep using your oven, but most of the equipment can be stored in regular closets, cabinets, or on shelves. The dehydrator can sit on the washing machine or dryer without any inconvenience, if you have a front-loading type. Sprouts can drain right in the sink or on the porch (either in bottles or in a plastic dish drainer) so that they can be moved about when necessary.

For the actual food preparation, you will need plenty of counter space. A covered table top will do. It may also be helpful to use plastic bags for garbage if you cannot compost, and do not have a disposal. Rejuvelac, often used in recipes or alone, can be stored in jars in the refrigerator while other bottles are being prepared somewhere in the kitchen or pantry. A piece of cheesecloth covering the jars will protect their contents. Prepared seed cheeses and yogurts can be placed in a jar (covered with a cloth or towel) next to the Rejuvelac or on top of the refrigerator. The warmer the place where you put fermented preparations, the less time will be needed to complete the process. The same goes for hotter climates and summer weather versus colder climates and cooler indoor temperatures.

Things To Have On Hand

There are many frequently used foods—I call them basics—that are good to have on hand always. All the sprouting seeds, grains, and beans should be regularly replenished and placed in labeled plastic or glass jars with lids. Wheatberries for planting, sprouting, and use in recipes, hulled and unhulled buckwheat for sprouting and planting, and unhulled sunflower seeds for greens can be purchased in bulk (see Appendix B for information about suppliers) and are best stored in a dry, cool place in plastic or glass containers or inside plastic bags in a covered barrel. Hulled sesame and sunflower seeds, raw almonds, and other nuts are also good to keep in stock.

Dried and fresh fruits should also be plentiful in your kitchen. Try a variety of dried (unsulfured, natural) fruits, especially in the winter when ripe fresh fruits are expensive and scarce. Fruits bought unripe that will ripen off the tree or vine include apples, pears, some melons, apricots, avocados, plums, peaches, tomatoes, mangoes, and bananas. These can be placed in a paper bag to speed up the process. Fruits that will not ripen are pineapples, grapes, citrus fruits, small melons, and berries—these should not be used if unripe. Chances are that they are out-of-season and expensive if unripe, anyway. Ripe fruits can be stored in the refrigerator, peeled and pitted and frozen for later use, or dehydrated and resoaked when needed.

A variety of fresh vegetables should be bought frequently and those that will not be eaten that day placed in the refrigerator in glass or plastic containers. Refrigeration tends to extract the moisture from foods, leaving them dry and limp unless they are kept covered. This is especially true for sprouts, greens, lettuce, and fresh herbs. As with fruits, excess or unused vegetables can be cut and dried for later use in soups or as vegetable chips.

Condiments

The judicious use of seasonings can enliven any recipe. The condiments that are recommended for use on the Hippocrates Diet include certain herbs and spices, sea salt, lemon juice, and raw honey. These condiments provide a variety of flavors.

Many herbs and spices have medicinal value, but for culinary purposes they all should be used in small amounts.

Herbs	**Spices**	**Aromatic Seeds**
Bay leaf	Allspice	Anise
Basil	Cayenne	Cardamom
Chives	Cinnamon	Caraway
Dill	Clove	Celery seed
Marjoram	Curry	Coriander
Mint	Ginger	Cumin
Oregano	Mace	Dill
Parsley	Nutmeg	Fennel
Rosemary	Orris root	Mustard
Sage	Paprika	Poppy seed
Tarragon	Saffron	
Thyme	Vanilla	
Yarrow		

If you use salt, it is best to use it in the form of tamari or miso (both are fermented soy products which contain about 20 percent sea salt, and valuable food enzymes), one of the various vegetable salt substitutes, or kelp powder. Lemons are another flavoring you might want to have on hand regularly. Try to get tree-ripened or organically grown lemons if possible. Powdered or fresh onion and garlic may be too stimulating for people with digestive problems, and should be avoided by those people.

For family members who use vinegar, apple cider vinegar is best. It can be mixed with water and added to the new oil-free packaged salad dressings available at natural foods stores. For yourself, lemon juice and water may be added. Always check the ingredients in salad dressings before buying them—many supermarket brands contain preservatives. Many of the oil-free dressings taste quite good and can be used for company—if you are in a hurry—or if you don't have the ingredients on hand to make one of the fresh dressings on page 128.

One final ingredient to have on hand is uncooked, unfiltered honey. It may come in a semi-hardened or crystallized (whitish) form. To liquefy it, merely place the jar in warm water for an hour or so. Do not store it in the refrigerator or it will harden again quickly. Raw honey is good added to cereals, seed yogurts, Rejuvelac, seed milks, fruit salads, and desserts. Because it is a concentrated source of simple sugar, it is best used in small quantities, especially by those with serious health problems such as hypoglycemia.

Now that you have all your essentials, let's go right on to the details of live food preparation and the recipes.

HIPPOCRATES DIET RECIPES

At last, here's what you've been waiting for! Perhaps you have just picked up this book, skipped all the rest for now, and want to put the Hippocrates Diet right into practice. That's great! The only introduction this section needs is a smile, a paperweight, and a hand. The smile is for you, the paperweight is to hold the pages open, and the hand is what I hope I can give you while you prepare your first live food meal. The recipes in this section are long-time favorites of mine. The proportions listed serve two to four people, and you can vary them according to the size of your family.

A meal of salad and bread or soup will take about twenty minutes to prepare. Preparation time may vary up to an hour, as for an unusually large meal of soup, sprout loaf, salad, and dessert. Have fun—and remember, the real proof of what I say is in the pudding (or putting)—your putting live food on the table and in your body, every day.

BASIC RECIPES

These basic recipes are the ones that you will need to know how to make in order to prepare many of the other recipes listed. Sauerkraut, Rejuvelac, Seed Cheese, and Seed Yogurt are also tasty without accompaniment, and should be used frequently.

Nut Butter

---

2 cups shelled raw almonds *or* hulled raw sunflower seeds

Run nuts or seeds through Champion Juicer with the "homogenization blank." If you do not have a Champion Juicer, use a setting that will finely grind the seeds or nuts without separating out the oil. Store unused nut butter in a glass jar in the refrigerator.

Rejuvelac

½ cup 24-hour sprouted soft pastry wheat-berries (available at natural foods stores)
spring or filtered water

Grind wheatberries and put ¼ cup each in 2 large jars. Fill jars almost to top with water and cover with cheesecloth and an elastic band. Allow the mixture to sit for 3 days. On the fourth day, pour off Rejuvelac, straining out berries and sediment. Store unused

Rejuvelac in the refrigerator. It will keep several days. Start a new batch twice a week.

Sauerkraut

- 2 large heads cabbage, green and/or red
- 2 beets, trimmed and grated (optional)
- 7 juniper berries, ground (optional)
- 4 teaspoons dulse *or* wakame, soaked and chopped (optional)
- 1 teaspoon kelp powder (optional)
- 1 teaspoon dried dill or 2–3 teaspoons fresh (optional)

Grate cabbage and save 2 or 3 outer leaves. Place cabbage, beets, and other ingredients in a bucket or pail till half full, and with a bat or 2″ × 4″ board, pound cabbage mixture firmly until it becomes juicy. The more you pound, the better. Place pounded mixture in a crock, glass bowl, jar, or stainless cookware, and cover completely with outer leaves. On top of leaves, put a plate and a brick or heavy stone to weigh them down. Next cover the crock itself with a cloth or towel and set it in a warm place. Leave undisturbed for 6–7 days. After 7 days, remove the weight and discard exposed leaves. Skim mold and residue from the top layer. Underneath you will find fresh, tasty sauerkraut. Place kraut in glass jars and cover securely with lids. It will keep in the refrigerator for 3–4 weeks.

Seed Cheese

- 1 cup Rejuvelac (see page 110) *or* spring or filtered water
- 1½ cups hulled raw sunflower seeds
- ½ cup hulled raw sesame seeds

Soak seeds 8 hours and sprout for 8 hours. After this time, pour Rejuvelac into a blender. Blend at high speed, slowly adding seeds until all are blended to a smooth paste (approximately 4 minutes). Pour the mixture into a glass jar, cover with a cloth or towel, and set aside for 4–8 hours. If Rejuvelac is not available, use water and let mixture sit 2 extra hours. Or, save 1/4 cup from a previous cheese culture and mix it with the new batch. After the 4–8 hours have elapsed, pour off the whey by inserting a wooden spoon down one side of the jar to form a tunnel and spilling the liquid into the sink. This recipe yields approximately 2 1/2 cups of cheese. Store it tightly covered in the refrigerator. Refrigerated, the cheese will last 5 days.

Seed Yogurt

---

2 cups Rejuvelac (see page 110) *or* spring or filtered water
1 1/2 cups hulled raw sunflower seeds
1/2 cup sesame seeds

Follow the same procedure as for Seed Cheese (above), only set mixture aside for no more than 6 hours. Stir and refrigerate. This recipe yields about 4 cups.

See also: *Moo-less Milk,* page 115, *Basic Bread,* page 136, and *Basic Uncooked Pie Crust,* page 142.

BEVERAGES

These recipes for juices and other beverages include many combinations of fruits, greens, and vegetables that go well together. Yet many of these can also be used straight. Carrots, grapes, apples, oranges, grapefruits, tomatoes, and some other fruits and vegetables taste great by themselves, while parsley, beets, celery, spinach, and lettuce are too strong-tasting to be used alone.

When juicing any fruit or vegetable, be sure to cut it into pieces small enough for your juicer to handle. For example, an apple may be cored and cut into quarters. If you have any questions, refer to the manufacturer's instructions. You can leave the peels on, as the juicer will separate them out during juicing. To strain out any indigestible pulp or fiber that is not separated from the juice by the juicer, pour the fresh juice through a wire mesh (preferably stainless steel) strainer.

When blending fresh fruits like peaches, apples, and pears for smoothies and shakes, it is best to peel them first. Since some of the most important nutrients are close to the skin, try not to remove any fruit along with the peel. Always remove the pits or cores.

Fresh juices begin to lose their nutritional value immediately, and therefore the maximum storage time is one day in the refrigerator. The exception is wheatgrass, which is even more volatile, and therefore should be discarded if not used after 12 hours.

Almond Frappé

---

2 cups Moo-less Almond Milk (see page 115)
1 tablespoon raw honey
½ cup banana ice cream (see page 144)
natural vanilla extract

Place first three ingredients and a dash of vanilla extract in a blender. Blend at medium speed for about one minute or until frappé is smooth in texture. Serve immediately.

Apple-Carrot-Beet Juice

---

2 large apples, washed and cored but not peeled
  (to yield about 2 cups fresh juice)
1 large beet, washed and trimmed but not peeled
  (to yield about ½ cup fresh juice)
8–10 medium carrots, washed and trimmed
  but not peeled (to yield about 3 cups fresh juice)

Cut apples and beet into pieces. Juice with carrots in high-speed juicer. Strain out pulp using wire mesh strainer, and serve.

Banana Milkshake

2 large bananas, peeled, frozen, and
chopped (to yield approximately 1 cup)
5 cups Moo-less Milk (see page 115)
natural vanilla extract

Place bananas, milk, and a dash of natural vanilla extract in a blender. Blend at medium speed for about 1 minute or until mixture is smooth and creamy. Serve.

Berry Delicious

4 fresh oranges (to yield about 2 cups fresh juice)
1 pint fresh strawberries
1 cup spring or filtered water

Squeeze oranges until you have 2 cups of juice. Wash strawberries, remove tops, and place berries in a blender with juice and water. Blend at medium speed for about 1 minute or until mixture is smooth. Serve.

Carrot Juice

12 medium carrots, washed and trimmed but
not peeled

Juice in high-speed juicer and serve. Yield is approximately 4 cups fresh carrot juice.

Grasshopper

$\frac{1}{3}$–$\frac{1}{2}$ pineapple (to yield 2 cups fresh juice)
$\frac{1}{2}$ cup spring or filtered water
$\frac{1}{4}$ cup wheatgrass juice
4 leaves fresh mint (optional)

Place all ingredients in blender. Blend on high setting until smooth (about 1 minute). Strain through a wire mesh strainer to remove pulp, and serve immediately.

Green Drink

4 cups sprouts (adzuki, alfalfa, cabbage, lentil, mung bean, or wheat)
4 cups buckwheat and sunflower greens
5 medium carrots, washed and trimmed but not peeled, and cubed (about 3 cups)
5 large celery stalks (about 3 cups)
1$\frac{1}{2}$ medium cucumbers (peeled if waxed), cut into pieces (about 3 cups)

Juice ingredients in a wheatgrass (slow-turning) juicer. Strain through a wire mesh strainer to remove pulp, and serve immediately. This recipe yields 8 ounces of juice.

Moo-less Milk

1 cup (pressed) wheat sprouts, *or* 1 cup soaked raw almond, sesame, or sunflower sprouts
5 cups spring or filtered water

Place sprouted seeds, wheat, or nuts and 1 cup of water in a blender. Blend at medium speed until mix is paste-like. Add the rest of the water and blend at high speed for 2 minutes. Strain out the pulp with a wire mesh strainer and discard. Store milk in a glass jar in the refrigerator for up to 4 days. Add to other recipes as directed. This recipe yields approximately 5 cups.

Peaches 'n' Cream

- 2 large ripe peaches
- 1 banana
- 2 cups Moo-less Almond Milk (see above)

Peel peaches and banana, cut into pieces, and place in blender. Blend at medium speed for 1 minute or until smooth. Serve immediately.

Spicy Green Drink

- 4 cups buckwheat greens
- 4 cups sunflower greens
- 4 cups alfalfa sprouts
- ⅓ head lettuce *or* 2 cups other green leafy vegetables
- 3 celery tops
- 1 red pepper, seeded and sliced
- 1 large scallion
- 1 small bunch parsley
- 4 tablespoons Sauerkraut (see page 111)

Measure leafy greens by pressing them into a measuring cup. Wash all vegetables thoroughly and then juice them in a slow-turning juicer. Strain out pulp by pouring juice through a wire mesh strainer, and serve immediately.

V-5

- 3 large celery stalks (to yield about 1 cup juice)
- 6 large carrots, washed and trimmed but not peeled (to yield about 3 cups fresh juice)
- 1 cup alfalfa sprouts
- 1 tomato, sliced
- 1 dash tamari (natural soy sauce)
- 1 small bunch parsley (optional)

Juice celery and carrots in high-speed juicer. Blend the juice with the other ingredients in a blender at high speed until the sprouts, tomato, and parsley are liquefied. Serve V-5 immediately with celery sticks.

Watermelon Juice Cooler

- 6 cups watermelon chunks (including rind and seeds)

Juice all parts of the watermelon in a high-speed juicer. Serve with additional chunks of red watermelon.

Wild Weed Drink

- 2 cups young dandelion greens
- 2 cups lamb's-quarter tops
- 2 cups purslane
- 1 red pepper
- 2 large carrots, washed and trimmed but not peeled
- 2 tablespoons Sauerkraut (see page 111)

Press greens into a measuring cup to measure. Remove stem and seeds from red pepper, and slice. Juice ingredients in wheatgrass juicer. Serve immediately.

See also: *Rejuvelac,* page 110.

SOUPS

Refreshing, light, and easy to digest, raw soup is a delightful addition to any Hippocrates Diet meal. Serve soup with salads, grain crisps, and full-course meals. Or make soup in the morning, put it into a Thermos container, and have it for lunch with some avocado sliced into it.

Soups are quick and easy to make. As a base they use vegetable or fruit juices blended with other ingredients. Since the ingredients remain raw, these soups do not keep as long as cooked soups, and therefore you should discard leftovers.

Quick Vegetable Soups

Blending techniques for vegetable soups vary. If the soup is somewhat chunky, as with Gazpacho, the blender should be set on a slow speed for about one minute. For a creamy soup, blend at medium-high speed for two minutes or so until the soup reaches the desired consistency.

During the winter you may use warmed, but not boiled, water where water is required in preparing the soups. Alternatively, you may pour the soup into a heat-resistant glass container and place it in hot water until it is warmed. This will prevent direct contact with the heat source, and preserve the enzymes in the soup.

When you use avocados in these recipes, cut them in half, remove the pits, and scoop the meat out of the peels with a spoon. Discard the peels. If the meat won't scoop out easily, the avocado is not ripe yet. (Ripe avocados "give" when you press them with your thumb.) Use only ripe avocados in these recipes.

Carrot Soup

6 medium carrots, washed and trimmed but not peeled (should yield about 3 cup fresh juice
1 cup shelled whole walnuts, soaked 6 hours in 2 cups spring or filtered water
1 small zucchini
1 teaspoon tamari (natural soy sauce) *or* kelp powder
½ teaspoon ground caraway seeds

Juice carrots in high-speed juicer. Blend with other ingredients in a blender at medium-high speed until soup has a creamy consistency. Serve with alfalfa sprouts and Grain Crisps (see page 137).

Corn Chowder

1 large avocado
6 ears fresh corn, cut off cob
spring or filtered water
1 tomato, sliced (optional)
1 cup mixed vegetables, diced
½ cup (pressed) dulse

Soak dulse in spring or filtered water for a few minutes. In the meantime, peel avocado, scoop out pulp with spoon, and place in blender with corn, water, and tomato. Blend on medium speed for 2 minutes or until chowder is smooth in texture. Drain and chop dulse. Stir in diced vegetables and dulse, and serve with a salad.

Gazpacho

2 medium tomatoes, cubed (about 2 cups)
1 cup alfalfa sprouts
½ lemon, juiced
½ avocado
1 celery stalk
1 scallion
1 pinch basil (fresh or dried)
1 pinch oregano (fresh or dried)
1 teaspoon tamari (natural soy sauce)
1 dash cayenne (optional)

Place ingredients in a blender and blend at low speed for 1 minute. Soup should retain a slightly chunky texture. Serve with Grain Crisps (see page 137).

Indian Cucumber Soup

2 large cucumbers, peeled and chopped
1 cup Seed Cheese (see page 111)
¼ cup chopped parsley
1 scallion
½ teaspoon cumin powder
spring or filtered water

Place first five ingredients in blender and blend at medium speed, adding enough water to obtain a soup consistency. Serve with your favorite loaf.

Spinach Soup

1½ cups (pressed) spinach
1 medium tomato, chopped (about 1 cup)
½ avocado
1 teaspoon tamari (natural soy sauce) *or* kelp powder
1 cup Rejuvelac (see page 110) *or* spring or filtered water

Blend ingredients in a blender at medium-high speed until smooth. Serve with Basic Bread (see page 136).

Fruit Soups

These smooth, thick fruit soups are often served in place of a vegetable meal at the Hippocrates Institute. They are best eaten alone or with a fruit salad, and they make an excellent breakfast. They do not mix well with vegetable meals.

When blending whole fruits to make these soups, wash, peel, and cut the fruits first. If the fruits are organically grown, you may use the peels if you wish. Fresh fruits may be frozen while they are in season, but they should be used within a month or two.

When soaking dried fruits for use in soups, wash them and soak them until they are soft. You may find it convenient to leave them overnight. I like to keep a variety of soaked dried fruits in the refrigerator at all times. Dried fruits will keep for up to a week in water in the refrigerator.

Be sure to remove the pits from prunes, apricots, and any other unpitted dried fruits you buy. Raisins and figs have small edible seeds instead of pits, and some types of dried fruit are sold already pitted.

Cantaloupe Soup

1 small or ½ large cantaloupe, peeled and cut (about 4 cups)
½ teaspoon powdered ginger

Place cantaloupe pieces and ginger in a blender and blend at medium speed for 1–2 minutes or until smooth and creamy. Serve.

Golden Fig Soup

1 banana, peeled and cut
2 cups dried calimyrna figs, soaked overnight in 3 cups spring or filtered water
water from soaking figs
spring or filtered water (cool or warm)

Place fruit together with fig soak water in a blender and blend at medium speed for 1 minute or so. Add 1–2 cups more water to make a creamy soup. Continue blending (about 2 minutes in all). Try substituting dried black mission figs or dried apricots for variety.

Grape and Nut Soup

½ cup shelled walnuts
1 small bunch seedless grapes
1 large apple, peeled, cored and chopped (about 1 cup)
1 cup fresh apple juice (approximately 1 large apple)

Soak shelled walnuts for 6 hours or overnight. Chop the walnuts fine. Blend ingredients in a blender at medium speed for about 2 minutes or until smooth.

SALADS

Vegetable and sprout salads are mainstays of the Hippocrates Diet. You should eat a salad composed of a variety of fresh sprouts, greens, and vegetables twice each day on both the cleansing and the building/maintenance diets.

If you use the finest whole ingredients available, and experiment with these recipes, you will soon discover how satisfying a living foods diet can be. Use the delicious salad dressings listed on pages 128–130 for added zest.

Vegetable and Sprout Salads

When choosing greens, lettuce, and other vegetables for use in salads, be sure to get the freshest and tastiest ones available. If possible, get organic vegetables or grow your own garden. The greens you use should be crisp, the carrots and broccoli snappy. Cucumbers, celery, and sweet peppers should be purchased unwaxed, firm, and fresh. Hothouse or non-vine-ripened tomatoes should be used sparingly or avoided altogether. Wash all vegetables before using them.

If a recipe calls for grating, cutting or dicing that can be performed by your food processor, use it. Otherwise a sharp knife and a cutting board will do. All ingredients for the salads, except lettuce and greens, should be cut into bite-sized pieces, unless otherwise directed. Generally, lettuce and greens such as spinach, Swiss chard, buckwheat, and sunflower should be broken up into bite-sized pieces by hand. This way, leftover salad greens won't turn brown.

Complete Meal Salad

1 cup alfalfa sprouts
1 cup sunflower greens, torn in half
1 cup mung bean sprouts
1 cup greens, torn into small pieces
¼ summer squash, grated
1 avocado, cubed
½ cucumber (peeled if waxed), sliced
1 tomato *or* 1 red pepper, seeded and diced
1 teaspoon kelp

Toss all ingredients together and serve with your favorite homemade dressing.

Garden Salad

2 cups spinach, torn into small pieces
1 cup alfalfa sprouts
½ cup cabbage sprouts
1 cup thinly sliced romaine lettuce
½ cup thinly sliced red cabbage
2 small carrots (washed and trimmed but not peeled), thinly sliced (about ½ cup)
2–3 radishes, thinly sliced (about ¼ cup)
1 medium tomato, sliced

In a large serving bowl, toss all ingredients except for tomato. Place tomato slices around top.

Hippocrates Salad

2 cups chopped sunflower greens
2 cups chopped buckwheat lettuce
2 cups alfalfa sprouts
1 cup lentil or mung bean sprouts
1–2 celery stalks, chopped (about 1 cup)
3 red peppers, seeded and chopped (about 1 cup)
2 tomatoes, cubed (about 2 cups)

Toss all ingredients together and serve with your favorite homemade dressing.

Oriental Sprouts and Vegetables

1 cup fenugreek sprouts
1 cup mung bean sprouts
1 cup adzuki sprouts
1 red pepper, seeded and cubed (about ½ cup)
1 medium celery stalk, chopped (about ½ cup)
½ cup snow peas, chopped with pods
½ cup Chinese cabbage, chopped
¼ cup scallions, diced
2 cloves garlic, pressed
1½ cups spring or filtered water
¼ cup tamari (natural soy sauce)
½ lemon, juiced

Marinate vegetables (including the scallions and garlic) and sprouts in water, a little tamari, and lemon juice for 2–4 hours. Serve with small cubes of avocado on a bed of buckwheat greens.

Salad Rolls

2 cups alfalfa sprouts
1 cup mung bean sprouts
1 large tomato
1 avocado
1 dash tamari (natural soy sauce)
10 outer leaves romaine lettuce *or* 4 sheets nori sea vegetable

Mix sprouts with tomato and avocado pulp, add tamari, and roll inside lettuce leaves or nori sheets. Serve.

Sea Salad

¼ cup (pressed) dulse sea vegetable
¼ cup (pressed) arame sea vegetable
2 cups lentil sprouts
¼ cup chopped scallions
1 medium celery stalk, chopped (about ½ cup)
½ avocado, chopped (about ½ cup)
½ lemon, juiced

Soak sea vegetables for a few minutes, drain, and chop. Mix with lentil sprouts, chopped scallions, celery, and avocado, and sprinkle juice of ½ lemon on top. Serve.

Watercress Salad

1 cup watercress
1 cup buckwheat greens
½ cup lentil sprouts

1 medium celery stalk, chopped (about ½ cup)
1 avocado, cubed (about 1 cup)
1 lemon, juiced

Measure the greens by pressing them into a measuring cup. Tear them into bite-sized pieces. Toss with lentil sprouts, chopped celery, and avocado cubes. Sprinkle with lemon juice and serve.

Fruit Salads

In preparing fruit salads, where the whole ingredients are very visible and retain their individual flavors, it is very important to use the freshest, ripest fruit you can find. Buy red cherries, not pink ones, and soft peaches instead of hard. Bananas should be eaten when they are sweet—when all traces of green have disappeared. Grapes should be red, purple, or yellow-green (depending upon the variety) when they are ripe and sweet. Pineapple should be golden brown when you use it. And so on.

Fruit salads are best with fruit soups, as a light meal with fruit sauces, or on their own.

Citrus Salad

---

2 oranges, peeled and sectioned
1 grapefruit, peeled and sectioned
⅛ fresh pineapple (about ½ cup chopped)
⅓ pint strawberries, without tops
1 cup shelled raw almonds (about 1 cup almond powder)

Cut fruits into bite-sized pieces and mix in bowl. Powder almonds in seed or nut mill, sprinkle on top of salad, and serve.

Northern Salad

½ cup dried pitted apricots
½ cup fresh blueberries
1 cup shelled raw pecans, chopped
2 medium apples, peeled, cored, and chopped
1 large pear, peeled, cored, and chopped
1 tablespoon raw honey (optional)

Soak apricots until soft (about 6 hours) or overnight in 1 cup of spring or filtered water. Mix ingredients together, including 1 tablespoon of raw honey to sweeten if desired.

Tropical Salad

1 large mango (about 2 cups)
1 large papaya (about 2 cups)
1 medium banana (about 1½ cups)
1 cup grated coconut (fresh)

Peel and cube mango. Peel papaya, remove seeds, and cube. Peel and slice banana. Shape fruits into loaf and sprinkle with grated coconut.

SALAD DRESSINGS AND SAUCES

There are many delicious and healthy ways to make salad dressings and sauces for fruit salads. At the Hippocrates Institute, most salad dressings are based on avocados, sprouted seeds or nuts, seed cheese, or vegetables and their juices. Sauces for fruit salads consist primarily of sprouted seeds and nuts, fruits, and fruit juices. Of course, the fruit sauces should be used only on fruit salads, and the vegetable, avocado, or seed dressings on vegetable and sprout salads (see Food Combining chart on page 103).

Try to choose combinations of salads and dressings or sauces that go well together. Apple-Pear Sauce, for example, makes a poor accompaniment to Citrus Salad, but a good one to Northern Salad. Walnut-Carrot Dressing goes well with Sprout Salad or Garden Salad, but not so well with Sea Vegetable Salad. Other combinations are mentioned in the recipes, and you can try a few of your own.

Apple-Pear Sauce

1 large apple, peeled and cut into chunks
1 large pear, peeled and cut into chunks
½ cup pitted prunes, soaked overnight in 1 cup of spring or filtered water
water from soaking prunes
1 dash cinnamon
1 cup Rejuvelac (see page 110)

Blend fruit and cinnamon at medium speed in blender, adding fruit soak water and Rejuvelac until sauce is thick. Serve with Northern Salad (see page 128), or as a breakfast dish.

Avocado-Tomato Dressing

2 medium tomatoes, cubed (about 2 cups)
2 avocados
¼ cup chopped scallions
1 cup Rejuvelac (see page 110)

Place tomatoes in a blender and blend until liquefied. Then add avocado and other ingredients. Blend on medium speed until smooth. Serve with Hippocrates Salad (see page 125).

Blended Tomato Sauce

1 medium tomato, cubed (about 1 cup)
1 small garlic clove, pressed
¼ teaspoon basil

Blend tomato with garlic in a blender at low speed to make a chunky sauce for Italian Bread.

Company Sauce

1½ cups 1-day-old sunflower sprouts
½ beet, trimmed and sliced
1 scallion, chopped
2 cups Rejuvelac (see page 110)
1 teaspoon tamari (natural soy sauce)

Place ingredients in a blender and blend at medium speed until smooth. This dressing will last for 1 day in the refrigerator if there is some left over.

Lemon Mayonnaise Dressing

1 cup pine nuts, soaked for 6 hours in 2 cups spring or filtered water
1 lemon, juiced
1½ cups spring or filtered water *or* Rejuvelac (see page 110)
1 teaspoon tamari (natural soy sauce)
1 pinch garlic powder or 1 small garlic clove, pressed

Place all ingredients in a blender, and blend at medium speed until creamy, about 2–3 minutes. Pour over a salad of grated cabbage, carrot, and alfalfa sprouts.

Seed Dressing

1 cup Seed Cheese (see page 111)
½ scallion, chopped
½ medium red pepper, seeded and diced
½ medium cucumber (peeled if waxed), sliced
1 tablespoon tamari (natural soy sauce)
½ teaspoon kelp powder

Place all ingredients in a blender and blend at medium speed for about 2 minutes or until creamy and smooth. Serve with Complete Meal Salad (see page 124).

Walnut-Carrot Dressing

3 large or 5 medium carrots, washed and trimmed but not peeled
½–1 cup shelled raw walnuts, soaked for 6 hours in 1–2 cups spring or filtered water
1 scallion, coarsely chopped
1 teaspoon tamari (natural soy sauce)

Juice carrots. Pour juice into a blender and add other ingredients. Blend at medium speed until dressing is creamy. Serve with Garden Salad (see page 124).

ENTREES

The entrees listed are favorites at the Hippocrates Institute, where they are served along with large salads. You can also serve them with soups or by themselves.

Cauliflower Loaf

1 cup shelled dried almonds, soaked for 6 hours in 1½–2 cups spring or filtered water
1½ cups grated cauliflower
9–10 mushrooms, grated (about 1½ cups)
½ celery stalk, chopped
¼ scallion, diced
1 garlic clove, pressed
½ teaspoon dried basil
½ teaspoon dried ground sage

Grind almonds as finely as possible. Mix all ingredients well and shape into a loaf. Serve on a bed of lettuce with salad or soup. Garnish with parsley sprigs, if desired.

Croquettes

2 cups lentil sprouts
2 medium carrots, grated
1½ cups Seed Cheese (see page 111)
¼ cup diced scallion
¼ teaspoon cumin
1 garlic clove, pressed
½ teaspoon poppy seeds

Grind or mash lentils. Mix with all ingredients except poppy seeds. Shape mixture into croquettes and roll over poppy seeds. Serve with salad and dressing.

Guacamole Dinner

2–4 avocados, peeled and pitted
1 lemon, juiced
1 tomato, finely chopped
1 scallion, chopped
1 garlic clove, pressed
¼ cup mustard or radish sprouts (optional)
¼ teaspoon cayenne

Mash avocado and mix with other ingredients. Serve with your favorite salad.

Sprout Loaf

---

1 cup alfalfa sprouts
1 cup lentil sprouts
1 cup mung bean sprouts
½ cup cabbage sprouts
1 cup shelled raw almonds, ground
1 celery stalk, diced
1 scallion, diced
½ red pepper, seeded and diced
1 tablespoon tamari (natural soy sauce)

Mix ingredients in a bowl, adding just enough spring or filtered water to form a loaf. Serve on a bed of romaine lettuce.

Stuffed Peppers

3 cups 2-day-old chick pea sprouts
1 cup ground sesame seeds or ½ cup tahini (a sesame-based sauce)
1 lemon, juiced
1 celery stalk, diced
¼ cup finely chopped parsley
1 garlic clove, pressed
¼ teaspoon cumin
1 teaspoon tamari (natural soy sauce)
6 whole red peppers

Place all the ingredients except for the peppers in a blender and blend until thick and paste-like. To do this, you may have to shut off the blender for a while and stir the ingredients instead. Alternate blending and stirring until the mixture is thoroughly blended. The blade attachment of a food processor may work better. With a knife, scoop the seeds out of the peppers. Stuff the hollowed peppers and serve them with sprout salad. The stuffing can also be prepared as a dip for grain crisps and vegetables.

Sunflower Rolls

1 tomato (about ½ cup chopped)
2½ cups 1-day-old sunflower sprouts
1 lemon
1 teaspoon tamari (natural soy sauce), kelp, *or* dulse
1 cup alfalfa sprouts
1 small zucchini *or* yellow squash, diced (about 1 cup)
¼ cup diced celery
¼ cup diced scallion
6 sheets nori sea vegetable

Place tomato in a blender and blend until thoroughly liquefied. Add sunflower, lemon, and tamari, and blend on medium speed until smooth. Remove and mix with other ingredients in a bowl. Roll in sheets of nori sea vegetable. Pat edges of nori roll with a little water to make them stick. Place them on a serving plate with the seams downward, and serve surrounded by alfalfa sprouts.

Wheat Casserole

---

2 cups 2-day-old wheat sprouts
¼ cup dry unhulled sesame seeds, soaked 6 hours in ½ cup spring or filtered water
1 cup 1-day-old sunflower sprouts
1 cup shelled raw walnuts, soaked 6 hours in 2 cups spring or filtered water
1 zucchini
1 celery stalk, diced (about ½ cup)
1 teaspoon ground sage
1 teaspoon tamari (natural soy sauce)

In a food processor or blender, grind wheat, sesame, sunflower, and walnuts until mealy. Shred zucchini in food processor. Mix all ingredients together in a bowl and shape into a casserole. Serve.

See also: *Complete Meal Salad,* page 124.

BREADS, CEREALS, AND CRACKERS

Uncooked sprouted grain breads, crisps, cereals, and crackers provide calories and fiber to the Hippocrates Diet. The cereals make a great breakfast, while the breads and crisps are wonderful complements to salads, soups, or entrees.

Ideally, you should have a food dehydrator to make a steady supply of breads and crackers. The average time for drying breads in the oven is sixteen hours or overnight. In the sun, drying takes from twelve to twenty-four hours depending on the strength of the sun. But the sun doesn't shine all year round, and, to block out air pollution, bread must be kept covered while sun-drying. A dehydrator can cut drying times by as much as one half. So if you're committed to following the Hippocrates Diet, you should purchase a dehydrator. It will pay for itself in no time as it can also be used to dry fruits and vegetables during the local growing season, saving you the cost of storebought dried goods.

When oiling baking trays so that the dough doesn't stick, use unrefined olive or corn oil.

Basic Bread

---

4 cups 2-day-old wheat or rye sprouts
½ teaspoon ground caraway seeds

Grind, blend, homogenize, or food-process the grain. Add spice by hand and spread batter ¼-inch thick on an oiled tray. Cut batter into 3- or 4-inch squares before baking. Bake in the sun, a dehydrator, or an oven at less than 120°F. The bread is ready when it is dry and crispy.

Chick Pea Bread

---

2 cups chick pea sprouts
2 cups wheat sprouts
½ teaspoon cumin
1 garlic clove, pressed

Follow the same procedure as for Basic Bread (above) and serve with soup, salad, or Stuffed Pepper filling (see page 134).

Grain Crisps

2 cups 2-day-old rye or wheat sprouts
1–1½ cups spring or filtered water *or* Rejuvelac (see page 110)
½ teaspoon ground caraway seeds

Blend to the consistency of pancake batter and pour onto a cookie sheet or shallow baking dish. Bake in the sun or an oven under 120° F until dry and crispy. The thinner you pour the batter, the shorter the drying time.

Italian Bread

4 cups 2-day-old wheat or rye sprouts
½ tomato, chopped (about ¼ cup)
¼ cup pitted black olives
¾ red or green pepper, seeded and chopped (about ¼ cup)
½ teaspoon onion powder
½ teaspoon garlic powder, or 1 garlic clove, pressed
1 teaspoon basil, oregano, and thyme (any combination)

Grind, blend homogenize, or food-process the grain. Add other ingredients by hand and follow same procedure as for Basic Bread (see page 136). Serve with Blended Tomato Sauce (see page 130), chopped olives, or any other topping.

Lentil Bread

2 cups 2-day-old wheat sprouts
2 cups 2-day-old lentil sprouts
1 scallion, chopped
2 garlic cloves, pressed
½ teaspoon ground caraway seeds

Grind, blend, homogenize, or food-process the wheat and lentil sprouts. Add chopped scallion, garlic, and caraway seeds, and work into batter by hand. Place in sun or dehydrator, or bake in oven at a temperature less than 120° F.

Sprouted Wheat Cereal

½ cup raisins
2 cups (pressed) sprouted wheat
4 cups spring or filtered water
1 large apple, peeled, cored, and sliced, *or* 1 banana, peeled and sliced

Soak raisins in 1 cup of the spring or filtered water, for 1 hour or until soft. Reserve the water used in soaking the raisins. In a blender, blend wheat with fruit, water, and raisin soak water, at medium speed for about 2 minutes. Use warm filtered water if a warm cereal is desired. The Sprouted Wheat cereal should have a soupy consistency.

Sun Grain Cereal

1½ cups 2-day-old wheat sprouts
1 cup 1-day-old sunflower sprouts

½ cup pitted prunes, soaked overnight in
1 cup of spring or filtered water
water from soaking prunes
3 cups spring or filtered water

Place first 3 ingredients in a blender and blend at medium speed for 2 minutes, adding enough prune soak water with some of the 3 cups of spring water to obtain a soup-like consistency.

PUDDINGS AND OTHER DESSERTS AND SNACKS

Since fruits and vegetables are poor combinations at the same meal, it is best to wait at least one hour, and preferably two, between a vegetable-based meal and a fruit dessert. The puddings, desserts, and snacks listed below can tempt any sweet tooth without presenting the health hazards that accompany commercially produced goods baked with refined sugar, flour, and oils, but they are not recommended for use more than three to four times a week (unless you are trying to gain weight). For added variety when you do have desserts, try the many fruit beverages, salads, and sauces listed in other sections of this book.

Puddings

If you get tired of having cereal every morning, a serving of the Breakfast Pudding listed below is a marvellous way to stimulate your appetite. The other puddings are delicious any time of day, and they are easy and quick to prepare. For best results, these puddings should be blended on medium to medium-high speed for about two minutes. If there are leftovers, they will usually keep for one day in the refrigerator.

Breakfast Pudding

---

1 cup 1-day-old almond sprouts

½ cup dried figs, soaked until soft in 1 cup spring or filtered water
water from soaking figs
1 large apple, peeled, cored, and cubed
spring or filtered water

Blend sprouted almonds, figs, and apple cubes with fig soak water in a blender at medium speed. Add additional water as needed to obtain a soup-like consistency. For variation, try substituting hazel nuts or sprouted sunflower or sesame seeds (all soaked 6 hours or overnight) for sprouted almonds.

Carob Pudding

½ cup shelled raw almonds, soaked 6 hours or overnight in 1 cup spring or filtered water
2 bananas, sliced (about 3 cups)
½ cup raisins, soaked overnight or until soft in 1 cup spring or filtered water
water from soaking raisins
½ cup Rejuvelac (see page 110)
2 tablespoons carob powder

Blend all ingredients, including raisin soak water and Rejuvelac, in a blender at medium speed, adding carob last. The pudding should be smooth and creamy.

Creamy Apple-Walnut Pudding

---

1 apple, peeled, cored, and cut (about 1 cup)
2 cups dried apples, soaked 6 hours or overnight in 4 cups spring or filtered water
water from soaking apples
1 cup shelled walnuts, soaked 6 hours or

overnight in 2 cups spring or filtered water
1 tablespoon raw honey
cinnamon

In a blender, blend water from soaking apples together with fruit and nuts, adding honey and cinnamon to taste. Pudding should have a creamy consistency.

Tropical Blend

---

2 medium papayas, peeled and seed removed (cubed, about 3 cups)
1 medium avocado, peeled and pitted (cubed, about 1 cup)
1 teaspoon raw honey (optional)

Place papaya in a blender and blend until liquefied. At medium speed, blend in avocado and ½ cup spring or filtered water, adding raw honey if you wish. Tropical Blend should be very thick and creamy.

Desserts

If you are having company, you can serve these desserts with all the pride of an accomplished cook and with the added satisfaction that you are providing your guests with pies, cakes, candy, or ice cream that is as healthful as it is delicious.

Almond Bars

---

2 cups dried figs, unsoaked
1 cup grated coconut
1 tablespoon raw honey

1 teaspoon natural vanilla extract
½ cup shelled whole raw almonds

Grind figs in wheatgrass juicer, or chop them fine with a knife. Mix with coconut, honey, and vanilla. Place whole almonds along the top of each bar and chill in refrigerator for a half hour before serving. Leftover bars will keep for another day in the refrigerator.

Avocado Delight

---

4 apples, peeled, cored, and cut (about 4 cups)
1 large avocado
1 dash cinnamon

In blender, blend fruits and 1 dash cinnamon until creamy, adding ½ cup spring or filtered water if necessary to make blending easier.

Basic Uncooked Pie Crust

---

1 cup shelled raw almonds
1 cup dried figs, unsoaked

Grind almonds and figs in a seed and nut mill or wheatgrass juicer. Press into an oiled pie plate (use unrefined olive or corn oil), and add one of the fillings listed in this section.

Carob Banana Pops

---

4 firm bananas, peeled
10 tablespoons carob powder
5–10 tablespoons spring or filtered water

Mix carob powder with 5–10 tablespoons of water warmed just enough to dissolve the powder, to make a syrup. Stick a popsicle stick into each banana, and dip each banana into the syrup. Wrap popsicles in a piece of waxed paper and place them in the freezer overnight or until fruit is frozen. Pops will stay fresh about 2 weeks if they are kept covered in the freezer.

Coconut Banana Cream Pie

4 ripe bananas, peeled
1 cup grated coconut
½ teaspoon natural vanilla extract
1 Basic Uncooked Pie Crust (see page 142)

Mash bananas. Stir in coconut and vanilla. Fill pie shell and place pie in freezer for about 1 hour to set.

Fruit Cake

1 cup shelled raw almonds
1 cup hulled sunflower seeds
½ cup raisins, unsoaked
½ cup dried figs
½ cup dried pitted apricots
½ cup dried pineapple
½ medium banana, peeled (about ½ cup slices)

Soak almonds and sunflower seeds overnight in 1½–2 cups (each) spring or filtered water. Grind all ingredients together in a wheatgrass juicer or food processor. Press into an oiled loaf pan to form. Serve thinly sliced. Fruit Cake will keep in the refrigerator for 1 day.

Fudge

1 cup dried figs, unsoaked
1½ cups pitted dates
2 cups shelled almonds
1 cup shelled walnuts
¼ cup carob powder

Run fruit and nuts through a wheatgrass juicer or food processor, making sure all are mashed well. Mix in carob powder and spread batter in a shallow dish. Slice into squares and chill before serving. In the refrigerator, fudge will keep for 2 days.

Ice Cream

8–10 bananas, peeled and then frozen
1 mango, peeled, cut, and frozen (optional)

Run frozen fruit through high-speed juicer and serve immediately. Instead of bananas, you can blend frozen strawberries, blueberries, mangoes, or peaches a little at a time with good results. Peel and cut mangoes or peaches, and trim strawberries, before freezing them. Frozen fruits will keep in the freezer for up to one month, but ice cream will not keep.

Mango Pie

4 mangoes, peeled and chopped
½ cup raisins, unsoaked
½ cup shelled amonds, ground
1 avocado, peeled

½ lemon, peeled
1 Basic Uncooked Pie Crust (see page 142)

Fill pie crust with mixture of mangoes, raisins, and almonds. Mash avocado and lemon with fork and spread on as topping. If desired, chill before serving.

Pecan Pie

---

1 cup shelled pecans
1 cup dried figs, ground
1 large ripe banana, mashed (about 1 cup)
¼ teaspoon nutmeg
¼ teaspoon cinnamon
1 Basic Uncooked Pie Crust (see page 142)

Crush nuts, leaving a few whole for topping. Mix with ground figs, mashed banana, and spices. Fill pie crust and top with whole pecans. Chill for a few minutes before serving, if desired.

Snacks

These nutritious snacks will perk you up any time of day.

Sprouted Trail Mix

---

1 cup sprouted wheat
½ cup raisins
½ cup 1-day-old sunflower sprouts
½ cup shelled raw almonds
½ cup pine nuts

½ cup dried apples, chopped
½ cup dried pitted dates, chopped

Do *not* soak the fruits or nuts used in this recipe. Mix all ingredients. This Trail Mix should remain fairly moist. Store it in a glass jar in the refrigerator for up to 5 days.

Fruit and Nut Balls

---

1 cup pitted prunes
1 cup shelled walnuts
1 cup dried pitted pears
½ teaspoon natural vanilla extract
shredded coconut

Grind prunes, walnuts, and pears in a food processor or wheatgrass juicer until mixed well. Remove mixture and mix in vanilla by hand. Roll into balls. Roll balls in coconut, and either chill or serve immediately. Leftovers will keep for 2 days in the refrigerator.

Zucchini Chips

---

3 medium zucchini
½ cup tamari (or enough to cover zucchini chips)
paprika

Slice zucchini ¼-inch thick. Dip each slice in tamari (natural soy sauce) and sprinkle with paprika. Dry on flat glass sheets or baker's trays in sun, dehydrator, or low oven (under 120° F) until crispy. The zucchini chips will take about 16 hours in the oven or 12 hours in the dehydrator. (Times for sun-drying will vary.) Zucchini Chips may be stored in plastic bags at room temperature. For variety, try making chips from summer squash, carrots, tomato, or onion.

11

The Hippocrates Diet And Weight Loss

It's no fun being fat—no one knows that better than an obese person. It is estimated that nearly two of every three adult Americans are significantly overweight. And more than fifty million Americans are either dieting or are contemplating diets. We live in the mixed-up culture that worships slimness yet fosters obesity.

Screen star idols and famous athletes are slim and loved. "Stay slim!" screams the voice of society, "or risk being unwanted and unloved, even by your number one fan—you!" On the other hand, "You only go around once, why not grab for all the gusto you can. Live it up!" says the media advertising blitz aimed at seducing you to indulge once more in the "finery" of life—fattening food and drink. Unfortunately, it is practically impossible to stay slim on the kind of food that is served at restaurants and dinner parties. So we find ourselves voluntarily enlisting in one of the most dangerous wars in Western history, the war against fat.

For many Americans, the battle begins slowly. If out of the 2000 calories eaten per day, 40 of them are not burned and instead get stored in the body as fat, an extra 14 pounds of weight will be accumulated between the ages of 25 and 40. Theoretically, twenty minutes of slow walking or ten minutes of brisk walking every day could neutralize those extra calories. A change in food quality, with more whole vegetables, fruits, sprouts, and greens, replacing fattening foods such as butter, cheese, eggs, red meats, refined oils and sugar—would also work. Keep in mind you would have to start this preventive routine at twenty-five and continue it for life.

Obviously, not many people have practiced prevention and they are suffering for it.

It is no secret to see who is winning and who is losing the modern battle of the bulge, but why fight? Because being fat is psychologically crippling and physically menacing. Dr. Louis M. Orr, ex-president of the American Medical Association, was asked in a newspaper interview, "Do you consider cancer as the greatest threat we face?" He answered, "No. Cancer is the most dreaded disease in the United States. But the greatest danger to the health of the American people is obesity."

The medical consequences of obesity are not to be taken lightly. According to the Senate Select Committee's report entitled *Dietary Goals For The U.S.*, fat people do not live as long as lean people do and they are a lot less healthy while they are alive. Obesity increases the risks of developing diabetes, heart disease, hypertension, arteriosclerosis, gall bladder disease, and certain types of cancer. It aggravates gouty arthritis, damages the liver, increases the risk of hernias, and causes difficulty in pregnancy and childbirth.

Putting more food into the body than is needed results in stress to the heart and blood vessels. It slows blood and lymph circulation and causes blood pressure to rise. If you are a man between the ages of thirty-five and fifty, your chance of developing heart disease increases by 30 percent for each ten pounds above your ideal weight.

THE FAT INDUSTRY

The modern obesity epidemic has created a billion-dollar industry to fight fat. Health salons and reducing spas net more than $220 million; over-the-counter diet pills net $54 million; and dietetic foods more than $1 billion annually.

In bookstores, new diet books appear each week and sell millions of copies, despite the fact that all too often the diets themselves don't work, or have side effects that are worse than extra weight. The fight against fat has also spawned many bizarre and unnatural non-dietary medical techniques for treating the obese, especially the massively obese.

Some obesity specialists now resort to methods such as jaw-wiring, appetite-suppressant drugs, tying off part of the intestine, and stomach-stapling. In general, the non-dietary and dietary programs fail when the adherent returns to his former, fattening lifestyle.

In the years to come, the fat industry will probably continue to gain momentum. Most people play the diet yo-yo game, paying hundreds of dollars each year and risking their health on fad diets that allow them plenty of fattening foods, rather than following a sensible dietary program like the Hippocrates Diet.

THE HIPPOCRATES DIET AND WEIGHT LOSS

The Hippocrates Diet is high in carbohydrates, rich in vitamins and minerals, and low in fat, similar to the best working examples of modern weight loss plans (an example is the Pritikin diet). But the Hippocrates Diet has one outstanding feature—enzymes. It is a diet which is based on raw, clean and non-fattening foods, more so than any other diet. Most diets, even the best ones, fail to get results because of the absence of enzymes in them.

Cooked, enzymeless food is fattening, whereas the same amounts of raw food are not. This is true for animals as well as people. Modern farmers in the business of maximizing profit from farm animals have found that it is not profitable to feed cows or hogs raw potatoes because they "eat up the profits"—they don't get fat enough. Cooked potatoes—despite the added expense of cooking—produce fatter hogs and fatter profits. A similar thing happens to laboratory rats. On the ordinary scientifically balanced but enzymeless chow diet, lab rats put on weight at an alarming rate and develop many degenerative diseases. On a raw diet similar to the foods available in their natural environment, they maintain normal weight and resist illness. The same is also true for house pets. Modern pet food is enzymeless and causes obesity and a variety of diseases in our pets.

Almost fifty years ago, the researchers Kohman, White, Eddy and Sanborn, of Columbia University, used 1500 animals in an experiment comparing canned food diets with home-cooked and raw diets. The canned food was cooked at higher temperatures for longer times than the home-cooked food. The canned food eaters turned out to be the heavyweights, heading toward obesity quickly, and the raw fooders were lightweights. The researchers used the results to argue the increased absorbability of canned over home-cooked and raw food, suggesting that food is more nutritious after processing. It could also be argued that the raw food eaters, while maintaining balanced and normal weight and health, assimilated less food. But isn't the ideal function of food, to maintain normal weight and health? If cooked food causes obesity, aren't too many fat-inducing cooked calories being absorbed?

Judy Mazel, author of the popular book *The Beverly Hills Diet*, argues that fat is caused by "indigestion" of low-grade fuel. "When your body doesn't process food, doesn't digest it, that food turns into fat," says Mazel. "Your body, like an automobile, can only run on the fuel it's fed. If you put low-grade gasoline in a Rolls-Royce, it will soon need to be towed." But isn't weight gain really more a question of over-digestion and under-utilization of high-grade (overly concentrated) fuel, due to a sedentary lifestyle, wrong food choice and cooking? Mazel's answer is "conscious combining," a pseudo-scientific regime of binges (she calls this phase of the diet "open human") alternating with periods of "washing," "burning," "digesting" and "feeding" in which entire meals and days are devoted to eating certain fruits, allegedly endowed with gobs of enzymes. But on the whole, ripe fruits, except for bananas, mangoes, and avocados, and to a lesser extent figs and grapes, contain few active enzymes when compared with germinated seeds, grains, beans, and nuts. The enzymes in unpalatable green fruits such as pineapple and papaya are used by nature to ripen the fruit, and are not produced for human consumption. By the time these fruits are ripe, most of the enzymes in them have been used up.

HIGH-PROTEIN DIETS

It is not my aim to discredit the popular diet plans and their inventors, but I do feel that most of these diets are harmful to the body. Especially questionable are the high-protein diets, including the well-known Scarsdale, Atkins, and Stillman diets, although there have been others. These diets are predicated on the consumption of three times the normal amounts of lean beef and chicken—all high in protein—and they are not safe.

The high protein intake induces ketosis, a state of hyperacidity that is dangerous to the body. Toxic substances called ketones are formed as a result of overconsumption of proteins and fats and underconsumption of the carbohydrates needed to process fats. Ketosis can also be created by faulty carbohydrate metabolism, as is often the case in diabetics.

A high-protein diet stimulates dramatic, temporary weight loss. Large amounts of water are lost from the body tissues shortly after the diet is begun, as the body attempts to dilute the toxic byproducts of the excess protein ingested. Then weight is lost quickly with the elimination of the water and the toxins it carries out of the body. A week or so into the diet, the dieter hits a plateau. And when the diet is discontinued, the dieter gains weight rapidly. In Dr. Atkin's own words, "I concede that the worst feature about this diet is the rapidity with which you gain if you abandon it." But is it really the "worst" feature of the diet?

High-protein or liquid protein diets can cause kidney damage through ketosis; may bring on gout; may increase cholesterol and triglyceride levels, stressing the heart; may damage the liver; can cause constipation due to the excessive use of fiber-poor animal foods; can wash minerals and vitamins out of the body, causing tiredness, bone damage, and tooth decay; and increase the risk of certain types of cancer. Avoid them.

FASTING AND WEIGHT LOSS

Another popular weight loss scheme is fasting. Over the centuries, fasting has been used with reported success in treating a number of problems. For modern people and for weight loss, however, I believe it is dangerous and counterproductive. What we need today is nourishment and enzymes, not starvation. With the kinds of deficiencies many people are faced with today, prolonged fasting (taking nothing but water) if used widely, would probably result in more deaths than liquid protein diets. Without a steady supply of glucose from carbohydrates, the body turns to its own protein and fat to meet its energy needs. Protein is borrowed from tissues, muscles and organs, converted into glucose, and burned for fuel. By the end of a long fast, huge amounts of protein along with smaller quantities of fat, have been used by the faster's body for energy. The result can be a total weakening of the faster's organs and body tissues—damage that may take years to rebuild, and even then only if the maintenance diet used is adequate in vitamins, minerals, proteins, and enzymes for assimilation and carbohydrates for energy. Furthermore, after a fast, the body is more prone to weight gain due to its weakened condition.

The faster, like the high-protein dieter, alternates between his normal diet and "doing time," whether the "sentence" is eating lots of chicken or meat or fasting. But why bother fasting when a month of it may leave you only a few pounds lighter than a month of eating as much of the low-calorie Hippocrates Diet foods as you desire?

EXERCISE AND WEIGHT LOSS

Let's look at one more approach to weight loss that is popular today—exercise. Years ago, most people had to walk long distances to work and then do hard physical labor for hours each day. In the home, all sorts of chores were performed by hand which are done by machines today. Both men and women ate a diet which provided the majority of its calories from vegetables, grains, and fruits, with smaller quantities of animal foods. It's true today, as it was then, that those who work hard physically or exercise regularly, enjoy better health and a longer life. It is not true, however, that exercise is a substitute for a healthy diet.

Athletes and avid exercisers are still vulnerable to degenerative diseases and obesity. They enjoy better health and longer life than non-athletes because they fail to neglect only one important aspect of health, instead of two.

As a means of weight loss, exercise alone has not proven to be as effective as it is when combined with a sound weight loss diet, and it may be dangerous. Overweight people, especially heavyweights, are prime candidates for heart attacks produced by a prolonged, stressful exercise program. The excess fat on the body of a runner can work against the bones of his feet and back, making him accident-prone. If excess calories and wrong foods continue to stream into the body, even the ardent exerciser will hardly lose any weight. Chances are he will give up in time, due to lack of results for the amount of time spent.

When combined with the Hippocrates Diet, however, even light exercise like a brisk walk lasting one hour will help shed pounds. A brisk walk will burn 5.2 calories per minute, a total of 312 calories for an hour's walk. This is almost half the calories of a normal meal. At a more leisurely pace, 2.9 calories are used up each minute, for a total of 174 every hour. Exercise is indeed the dieter's best friend, not just because it burns calories, but also because physiologically, it is the fastest way to change metabolism, to cause a shift in the amount of food that is converted to energy rather than to fat. To convert food, and stored fat, to energy, we need the oxygen derived from exercise. Without it we feel tired and lazy because we cannot produce enough energy.

A half hour or more of brisk walking also stimulates the secretion of epinephrine (adrenalin), which helps to suppress the appetite. Jean Mayer, a renowned nutritionist, has shown how exercise such as walking actually reduces the need for food. Conversely, activity below a certain level increases this need. Whether you are overweight or not, it is a good habit to walk for an hour once or twice every day.

WHY WE GET FAT

As many causes have been offered for the problem of overweight as there are specialists, but the success of the Hippocrates Diet indicates that overeating of the wrong foods and underactivity are by far the most common causes. The change in the modern food supply (over the last one hundred years) is dramatic. The diet we eat today is high in fat, which has twice as many calories as proteins or carbohydrates. Simultaneously, processing has removed the low-calorie fiber and bulk from most foods—extracting the high-calorie parts of the plant for use as food. What is left is unbalanced, condensed, and fattening food—and an upsurge in obesity.

Yet the explanation that food and underactivity are to blame for the epidemic of obesity seems too simple, and for some reason unacceptable on a mass basis. Instead, many of us chase our tails—along with many experts who are lost in the jungle of extremely complicated physiological and psychological theories.

Some physiologists have argued that the thyroid is underactive in obese patients, using studies comparing people living inland with those by the sea (the former are more often iodine-deficient) to support their hypothesis. But throughout the entire United States, salt is iodized, and the fact is, hypothyroidism as a cause of weight gain is rare and can be treated easily. Other specialists have argued that the pituitary gland in fat people is abnormal, and that overweight people, failing to respond to the body's signals that hunger is abated, continue to eat. In rare cases, this may be true. However, for most of us, it is probably not.

Another theory is that the pattern of obesity is set in infancy—that an overfed baby is doomed to be a "fattie" for life. Dr. Jules Hirsh and his associates at Rockefeller University and Dr. Jerome Knitte of the National Institute of Health, among others, have measured the number and density of fat cells in infants in the first few months of life. Their results indicate that both the increase in the number of fat cells and their density in infants increase the risk of obesity in later life. Most people who have been fat since birth, however, have a normal number of fat cells, but an abnormal amount of fat in them. If you are one of these, you can easily achieve normal weight. There are rare cases of childhood obesity in which children become obese at an early age and have too many fat cells, but even this condition will eventually respond favorably to diet and exercise.

On the psychological side of weight loss, it has become "in" to treat obesity as a mental disturbance. But it's the old question of which came first, the chicken or the egg? Is it psychological trauma that begets obesity, or does obesity result in a lack of energy (laziness) and a poor self-image? Sure, there are rare cases where individuals have pathological food-related compulsions—but most fat people don't.

For all the emotionally charged causes (excuses) there are probably just as many factors that are overlooked, but the bottom line is this—we eat too much enzymeless, high-calorie, and fiberless food, and not enough uncooked, unprocessed whole fruits, raw vegetables, sprouts, greens, and grains. Processed foods are too dense in calories. If you use them, you can eat more calories at one sitting than is good for you, without realizing it. It takes thirty ears of corn to make the oil needed to fry an average serving of french fries. Two pounds of beets are needed to produce the sugar that flavors the fruit pie and soft drink in a typical fast-food meal. These items, and other over-refined and concentrated foods have less fiber to fill up space in your stomach than do foods in their whole state. You can eat more processed foods than whole foods (and get their extra calories) and still feel less full. Eating a balance of lower and higher-calorie whole living foods, you cannot fit enough food in your stomach in three satisfying meals to get fat! It's that simple.

HELPFUL WEIGHT LOSS IDEAS

At the Institute, I have worked with thousands of overweight people, nearly all of whom have had immediate weight reductions on the Hippocrates Diet. I am convinced that raw calories from uncooked foods are the key. Most of the raw fruits and vegetables used in salads are low-calorie foods. They do contain a marginal amount of enzymes, but are most important as rich sources of vitamins and minerals. A mistake that some people make is to eat plenty of low-calorie salads, but then turn to cooked foods to get the bulk of their calories. For best results, the majority of the calories in your diet should come from raw foods.

When trying to lose weight on the Hippocrates Diet, it is good to use some high-calorie raw foods like bananas, figs, grapes, avocadoes, sprouted grains, seeds, and nuts (and recipes made from them) each day. These foods are richly nourishing; they will fill you up, but not out. They will also supply you with plenty of energy.

These foods are also rich in enzymes for their efficient and total digestion in your body. The food enzymes in the Hippocrates Diet attack stores of fat and unwanted tissue, breaking them down cell by cell and eliminating them. As I discussed in Chapter 3, only enzymes can do the work of breaking up fat cells and eliminating their excesses. Raw foods and juices require less digestive juices from inside your body than do cooked foods. This allows your body's internal "house cleaning crew" to use all of its enzyme strength to break down and eliminate unwanted fat cells. This enyme strength is tied up by the digestive system of the cooked-food eater and is unable to help break down the excess fat unless the dieter literally starves himself. So on the Hippocrates Diet you can eat raw, fresh foods to your heart's content, and still lose weight safely and surely.

In order to maximize your weight loss, you can periodically eat mostly low-calorie raw foods, especially sprouts, greens, and cut vegetables in salads, with plenty of green drinks besides. A week every month will be often enough. But for the other three weeks of the month, follow the standard Hippocrates Diet, using all the different foods and food groups, including those higher in calories. The higher-calorie raw foods listed will be more satisfying and will add weight back if you find yourself getting too thin. In general, eat higher-calorie food to feel satisfied.

If you are overweight, with activity and walking each day, you should easily drop one to three pounds a week if you stick to the diet. Don't try to lose weight too rapidly, though. Shedding pounds too quickly can lead to loss of muscle and body protein, dehydration, acidosis, menstrual troubles, back pains, and hypoglycemia (low blood sugar). Eat! For breakfast have grain cereal, watermelon, dried prunes, or seed milk. At lunch eat a big salad with all kinds of sprouts, a seed, avocado or vegetable dressing, a handful of sprouted almonds and some basic bread with avocado spread. For dinner try soup, grain crisps, vegetable loaf, and occasionally, a piece of raw fruit pie. There's no need to make dieting a drag and starve yourself, when all it takes is a little creativity, time and effort to really enjoy your new diet.

Be sure to study Chapter 4 on cleansing the body. Remember, if all the doors are closed and you begin sweeping up the excesses in your body, you may feel rotten, and its nobody's fault but your own for letting yourself get that way in the first place. By keeping the eliminative channels open you will help make the diet a breeze, and you will gain more energy as you go without a bad day. Well, few bad days, anyway. There is bound to be a day or two when you feel famished and go off the diet.

If you do eat other foods or go out to eat, the next section should help you decide which foods to choose and why.

AT HOME, TRAVELING, AND EATING OUT

The content of this book, as you now know, is important to all of us. But it is "dead," like the pages it is printed on, if not put to use—just another academic exercise. It's not easy to make all the changes I recommend overnight, and it may not be healthy either. Unless, of course, you are fighting for your life against a chronic illness, and you must change quickly of necessity, a slower, more gradual change will be easier and better. Even so, only a thorough knowledge of the program and an unfailing desire to be healthier will help you stay on it, especially when cooking for the family, traveling or eating out.

Throughout this book, I have given numerous reasons and examples why the Hippocrates Diet works; why it is worth the effort to make it work for you; and what it will do. But nowhere have I mentioned how it will affect those around you—your family and close friends, and their opinion of your lifestyle.

Because you may be a little ahead of your time concerning diet and health, you can expect to make some of them feel a bit uncomfortable, especially at dinners and social or family gatherings. Not because you will be spouting out the theory of diet and health to your uncles, aunts, and friends, but simply because you will be practicing a healthy lifestyle. When the appetizers come around you might pass up Dotty's best crabmeat mushrooms or "pigs in a blanket," in favor of a plain carrot stick. When cocktails are served you may opt for straight tomato juice. During the main course you may eat vegetables and salad and no meat. Of course, all of this will arouse suspicion and sooner or later, you will allay all doubts by telling the others you are on a new diet.

Relieved, your friends will probably relate a few of their diet experiments—or stories of others they know who have had them—and they may even inquire about the diet you are on. Heaven forbid if you are already on the thin side! They might think you are too preoccupied with dieting, or even anorexic.

There is little doubt that occasionally a situation such as this one will present itself. And there are at least two ways to handle it. You can try to forget all that you know and pretend you eat just like everyone else, thus avoiding any uneasiness, or you can be yourself and make plans to notify people beforehand that you are on a special diet and would also like to bring something to eat with you. If you choose the first option after your body has been cleansed, it may not respond too well to the old foods and combinations of them. But for most people who are healthy to begin with, if they eat small amounts, nothing drastic will occur. It's what you eat every day that determines your level of health, not what is eaten on occasion.

Being yourself—doing your own thing—has great advantages. If your interest is in staying healthy and youthful, what's wrong with that? As long as dieters do not become dogmatic, experience has showed me that friends and relatives will learn from their example. Diet and health are "in," and the "laissez-faire" attitude toward health is on its way out. Self-responsibility in matters of health is now a strength and not a weakness. Openminded people will support you, listen to you, and may even try to practice a little of what you have to say. And the support you receive from interested friends and relatives will be invaluable to your emotional well-being.

Support from loving family members and children is wonderful, too. However, sometimes the changes are too great for your children or spouse to manage all at once. You need to take a patient and understanding approach. Asking them to try an occasional dish or to eat more vegetables may be a good start. You may even try putting out salad at every meal so they may eat some or not, as they desire. Certainly, removing foods containing additives and replacing them with comparable substitutes will cause little stir and may even be an interesting change. If your family rebels against anything you do, you may have tried too hard and, out of your love, pushed them temporarily in the opposite direction. But don't worry, they'll come around in time.

Occasionally, individuals will show up at the Institute who have been forced by a caring relative to come. From the first day (and sometimes to the last) they struggle and fight the simple ideas being lived and shared by the teachers and the guests. Enemas are "out of the question." Wheatgrass juice tastes "vile." The food doesn't fill them up—they wish they were home. No matter how much love and support the other students and staff show them, it is all "just so much bull."

For the most part, change hurts. It adds to the unpredictability and "human-ness" most of us fear. It presents new challenges and ideas we are unfamiliar with and demands a great deal of our energy when we must cope with it. And yet, though we often fight change to the end, it is inevitable and predictable because—everything is constantly changing. So why not stop fighting it and losing energy to it—and begin to accept, learn, and grow from it, as a tree learns to grow through a crack in the sidewalk rather than attempting to grow through the sidewalk itself.

It is obvious that some people we know are just not ready or willing to change, even if faced with the thought of a horrible disease. In such cases, I have found nothing more powerful then a good example—my own healthy lifestyle. Other people can see my energy and enthusiasm; my joy for living is never concealed, and there is a certain sparkle in my eyes. And so, in time, other people may let their guard down and begin making jokes about your peculiarities in eating. A few weeks later you may hear them telling friends what you have been hinting at all along. Soon after that, they might be seen secretively practicing a few health habits: avoiding fried foods; drinking less alcohol; eating more vegetables, fruits and salads; eating less meat and fatty cheeses; and refraining from late-night eating.

Who knows, the next time you come over, they may be serving an almost vegetarian meal for you and your family or other friends who are also beginning to adopt a healthier diet!

Traveling and Dining Out

Dining out with friends or while traveling will present new challenges also. Instead of frequenting the "old familiar" steak house or fast food establishment, you may choose to look for a good ethnic restaurant where salads and vegetarian dishes are available. At Italian restaurants, pasta, tomato sauce, vegetables and salad are available. Steamed vegetables and rice—ask for them without MSG (monosodium glutamate), please—are a good choice at a Chinese restaurant. Greek or other Mediterranian restaurants generally serve good salads and some vegetarian dishes. If you are satisfied with a good salad, you may find a soup and salad restaurant with a salad bar locally. In many cities, natural food restaurants are beginning to catch on. You can usually order a variety of salads, soups, and vegetables dishes at these.

If you are creative and bold enough to ask for what you want, in most cases, your meal will exceed your expectations. After all, you are paying for it. So be yourself and ask for what you want; without cheese; no oil; meatless; dressing on the side; steamed instead of fried, and so on.

When on the road, you may not always want to eat out. If you bring a small cutting board, bowls, forks and a small cooler chest with refreezable ice blocks (they can be placed in motel ice chests or freezers at night), you won't have to. You can make salads; sandwiches for the kids from raw vegetables, cheese, tomatoes, and whole wheat pocket bread; desserts from fruits and yogurt; snacks ranging from trail mix to carrot and celery sticks; and you can even grow sprouts in special travel sprout bags or jars. If you are going by car, most of what you need will be easy to bring along, and you may only need to stop occasionally at local produce stands or health food stores. If you are traveling by air, a sharp knife, forks, spoons, and a few dried seeds, nuts, and fruits for sprouting and eating will probably do. You can usually obtain plates and glasses wherever you are. You can soak seeds, nuts, and dried fruits in a glass with water overnight for breakfast the next day. In another glass, soak seeds to sprout in a sprout bag which you can hang in the shower or place inside a plastic bag in your car.

If you feel you need juice each day, you can bring along a fine grater and grate the vegetables or fruits and then squeeze the pulp and liquid through a sprout bag or cheesecloth. This will not work with wheatgrass, however, and if you cannot bring a hand juicer with you (most wheatgrass juicers can be operated either with a motor or by hand), the next best thing is a small meat grinder and a cheesecloth or strainer to press the juice from the grass.

If you plan to be on the road for an extended period, it is best to prepare ahead of time and experiment with sprout bags and travel accessories before you go. It also wouldn't hurt to contact one of the major vegetarian magazines such as *Vegetarian Times* or the *EastWest Journal* for a list of health and natural foods stores along your route. If you do happen to leave home totally unprepared, you can always ask people along the way where you can find what you need. If you go out of your way a bit to find alternatives, you will probably wind up meeting other people interested in health and getting some tasty vegetarian meals. When you arrive home, you will feel all the better for your efforts.

Remember, it's not what you eat occasionally that determines your level of health—it's what you eat every day that counts.

Epilogue

JOIN THE HIPPOCRATES DIET REVOLUTION

The Hippocrates Diet is indeed a revolution in diet, one which is needed desperately by people everywhere who have lost their sense of direction in matters of health. For years I have brought it to people all over the world, many of whom were suffering from depression or illness. The response has always been the same no matter where I present it—an eager "when can I begin?" Of course, some changes have to be made in your kitchen, your schedule, and perhaps most importantly, in your mind, before you can begin. But all of these changes add to the excitement and promise of what this journey to better health can bring.

Did you ever feel that you are missing something that you are having trouble pinpointing? At one time in my life I discovered that I was missing the vital live nutrients in raw foods, especially greens, green juices, Rejuvelac, sprouts, and wheatgrass. When I first noticed the power and energy they gave me, the way they balanced my body and banished a number of health problems I had, I knew I had made a discovery more powerful than all the medicines and other nutritional methods I had tried. Moreover, for the first time in my life I could amost completely control my diet and my health. It didn't happen overnight, of course, but as I became more sensitive, due to the cleansing nature of the diet and eliminative aids, a whole new sense of health and security came to me.

Have you ever felt completely in control of your health; clear and clean inside, full of energy, awake, confident, and relaxed? I can't promise that you ever will, but I do know that you can if you want to. As I mentioned in the very first chapter, all it takes is desire and a little effort—the diet and other health practices I recommend will take care of the rest.

If you are ready to escape the feelings of dependance and uncertainty you may have about your health; or if you are tired of learning to live with health problems, a lower-than-normal level of energy, or extra weight, give the Hippocrates Diet a try. If after a month you are not feeling 100 percent better, if you haven't lost that extra five to ten pounds, or if your energy level hasn't improved, go back and reread this book carefully. It is so different from your old way of life that you must first be sure to understand how it works and then follow my instructions properly. Otherwise your results will be mediocre at best.

I have tried my best to present the Hippocrates Diet and health program as clearly and simply as possible in this book. However, I know that it is not the same as being there with you in your kitchen to help you step by step. If you do have questions about the Hippocrates Diet that aren't answered in this book, or if after a second reading you are still having problems, call or write the Hippocrates Health Institute in Boston. Even better, make a reservation to come and learn the Hippocrates program first-hand with others who have come to do the same.

From the mountains of correspondence we receive, I know that nearly everyone who attends the Institute's two-week program finds it easy to stay on the diet almost entirely. Probably the most important reason is that they have practiced growing and preparing sprouts, greens, juices, Rejuvelac, and wheatgrass—all essential components of the diet.

The Hippocrates Diet is not a fruits, vegetables, and nuts diet. If you have read this far and think it is, reread this book from cover to cover; you have missed the essence of what I am saying. Sprouts, buckwheat and sunflower greens, Rejuvelac, fermented seed preparations, green drinks, fresh juices and wheatgrass are the foods that separate the Hippocrates Diet from any other ever proposed. Whereas fruits, vegetables, and nuts are important to the diet, they are incomplete by themselves.

The Hippocrates program is also incomplete unless you make an effort to exercise regularly, stretch, walk, breathe good air, get some sun, relax, spend time with good people, think positive thoughts, and do all the other little things that add up to a healthy lifestyle.

Before too long we will realize as a civilization what you have learned as an individual: your health is what you make of it. Everything you do and think either adds to the vitality, energy and spirit you possess or takes away from it. If you continually add to your lot, you will reap something much more precious than gold—you will reap perfect health and the peace of mind that accompanies it.

Appendix A

DAILY NUTRITIONAL NEEDS AND HOW THE HIPPOCRATES DIET MEETS (OR EXCEEDS) THEM

The proper quantity and quality of vitamins and minerals is essential to good health, especially when you are combating illness. Since all of the foods eaten in the Hippocrates Diet are uncooked, their full vitamin and mineral values are available to the body.

I have included a chart entitled *Essential Vitamins and Minerals—and What They Do*. In this chart, you will see the amount of each nutrient needed according to the recommended daily allowance (RDA) established by the U.S. government in 1980. The values given are for adult males (those for adult females are slightly lower). Alongside the RDAs you will find the estimated values of each nutrient supplied daily by the Hippocrates Diet. The Hippocrates Diet provides an adult with more than two times the RDA for almost every nutrient.

Following the Vitamin and Mineral chart I have included an *Estimated Nutritional Analysis of A Typical Hippocrates Diet Menu*, based on the United States Department of Agriculture (USDA) Handbook #8. A summary of the totals is included, indicating that the Hippocrates Diet contains more than six times the Vitamin C, two times the B-complex vitamins, ten times more Vitamin A, seven times more iron, five times the phosphorous, and two times the calcium of the RDAs. It also supplies nearly twice the protein with less than half the fat of the average American diet.

To increase or decrease the caloric value of the Hippocrates Diet, simply adjust your intake of the foods higher in calories. For example, to gain weight you can eat more breads, dried fruits, seed cheese, avocados, nuts, and bananas. To lose weight you can emphasize fresh vegetables, sprouts, leafy greens, juices, and certain fresh fruits.

Regardless of your aim it is important to use the green drinks. A glance at the Typical Menu chart reveals they are the most concentrated source of vitamins and minerals. In fact, green drinks are superior to many supplements because the nutrients they contain are chelated by nature. That is, they are found bound to other nutrients, exactly the way we have been getting our nutrients since time began. Supplemental vitamins and minerals, on the other hand, are a recent human invention and can create chaos in the body, especially when self-administered in larger doses than those found in foods themselves.

Indeed, the Hippocrates Diet provides super nutrition, safely, and at half the expense of other diets, including the one eaten by most Americans. As added protection we at the Institute also juice and drink wheatgrass juice, which I purposely haven't added to the charts (for a description of its nutrients see Chapter 8).

Some people mistakenly believe that wheatgrass by itself makes the Hippocrates Diet work. They continue to eat too much poor-quality food, thinking that the wheatgrass will balance it for them. This is not the case. By itself, wheatgrass will not work miracles; combined with the diet, however, it has been shown to be highly effective in cleansing the body and balancing overall health.

Following the Typical Menu chart, I have also included a handy *Composition of Foods* chart for easy reference to many of the foods commonly eaten on the diet.

ESSENTIAL VITAMINS AND MINERALS—AND WHAT THEY DO

Vitamins & Minerals	Food Sources	Function in Body	RDA (adult)*	Estimated Hippocrates Diet Value †
A (carotene)	alfalfa sprouts apricots carrots dandelion greens kale leafy greens orange and yellow vegetables peaches tomatoes wheatgrass	Aids normal growth, reproduction, and development. Aids skin, teeth, mucous membranes, and eyesight. Maintains resistance to infection.	5000 I.U.	30,000-50,000 I.U.
B_1 (thiamine)	alfalfa sprouts bean sprouts citrus fruits grain sprouts leafy greens nuts pine nuts sunflower seeds vegetables	Aids assimilation of starches and sugars; builds appetite and energy. Aids digestion, the heart, and the liver.	1.2-2.0 mg.	2.1-4.7 mg.
B_2 (riboflavin)	alfalfa sprouts almonds bananas citrus fruits kelp leafy greens mushrooms tomatoes soy sprouts sprouted beans and grains	Improves resistance to disease. Aids normal growth and development. Improves skin and eyesight.	1.6-2.6 mg.	2.7-3.97 mg.
B_{12}	bean sprouts dulse wheatgrass	Prevents nerve cell degeneration. Aids formation of red blood cells.	3-5 mcg.	5 mcg.

ESSENTIAL VITAMINS AND MINERALS, continued

Vitamins & Minerals	Food Sources	Function in Body	RDA (adult)*	Estimated Hippocrates Diet Value †
Niacin (a B vitamin)	alfalfa sprouts kelp leafy greens pine nuts sesame seeds sprouted beans and grains sunflower seeds tomatoes	Aids mental health and nervous system. Helps maintain appetite and adrenal health.	12-20 mg.	26-32.5 mg.
C (ascorbic acid)	cherries fruits kale leafy greens melons oranges and other citrus fruits parsley red peppers sprouts tomatoes wheatgrass	Aids growth and development. Maintains tissues, joints, ligaments, teeth, and gums. Promotes healing and resistance to infection.	75-100 mg.	300-418.8 mg.
D	almonds coconuts sunflower seeds sunlight	Promotes normal formation of strong bones and teeth.	400 I.U.	400 I.U.
E	beets celery leafy greens nuts and seeds oils sprouted grains wheatgrass	Aids reproduction, the heart, and the utilization of fatty acids.	10-30 mg.	20-45 mg.
K	alfalfa sprouts leafy greens sprouted grains	Aids blood coagulation. Decreases risk of hemorrhage in pregnancy.	—	—

ESSENTIAL VITAMINS AND MINERALS, continued

Vitamins & Minerals	Food Sources	Function in Body	RDA (adult)*	Estimated Hippocrates Diet Value †
Calcium	almonds dandelion greens dulse filberts kale kelp leafy greens nuts parsley sesame seeds and sprouts sprouts watercress wheatgrass	Builds healthy bones and teeth. Helps blood clot. Regulates heartbeat and mineral balance.	800 mg.	1500-2072 mg.
Chlorine	avocados celery kale kelp lettuce radishes red cabbage spinach tomatoes	Aids digestion and elimination. Sustains normal heart activity.	trace	trace
Iodine	dulse kelp leafy greens wheatgrass	Stimulates thyroid gland, which regulates rate of digestion. Important for growth and development.	—	.7 mg.
Iron	bean sprouts dulse fruits (dried and fresh) kelp leafy greens lentil sprouts nuts seeds	Helps form hemoglobin and myoglobin. Aids oxygen transport to cells and prevents anemia.	10 mg.	40-72.6 mg.

ESSENTIAL VITAMINS AND MINERALS, continued

Vitamins & Minerals	Food Sources	Function in Body	RDA (adult)*	Estimated Hippocrates Diet Value †
Phosphorus	bean sprouts dulse fruits kelp nuts pumpkin and squash seeds sesame seeds and sprouts sprouted grains sunflower seeds and sprouts vegetables wheatgrass	Builds and maintains bones, teeth, hair, and nervous tissue. Assists cells in absorbing fats and carbohydrates.	800 mg.	2500-4186 mg.
Potassium	bananas bean sprouts cabbage dried fruits dulse fruits leafy greens nuts wheatgrass	Maintains mineral balance and weight. Tones muscles. Aids disposition, promotes beauty.	—	14,452 mg.
Sodium	asparagus celery cucumbers dulse kelp olives sesame seeds and sprouts sprouts watercress	Aids digestion, speeds elimination of carbon dioxide, and regulates body fluids and heart action.	—	200-362.3 mg.

Abbreviations used in the above table:
I.U. — *International Units*
mg. — *milligrams*
mcg. — *micrograms*

Sources:
* RDAs: the figures used are adapted from the RDAs established for adult males by the U.S. Food and Drug Administration in 1980.
† Estimated nutritional content of the Hippocrates Diet (for one person, for one day) is based on *USDA Composition of Foods Handbook No. 8.*

ESTIMATED NUTRITIONAL ANALYSIS OF A TYPICAL HIPPOCRATES DIET MENU*

Food	Amount	Calories	Protein	Fat	Carbohydrate
Measurement Units			**Grams**		
Sprouted wheat cereal	1½ cups	198	5	.2	35.2
Banana	½ medium	51	.7	.1	13.2
Sprouted almond milk	¾ cup	100	2.7	6	1.4
Raisins	¼ cup	120	1	.1	32
Green drink	8 ounces	197	15.6	1.6	40.3
Hippocrates salad	1 serving	80	5.6	1.2	18
Seed dressing	½ cup	285	5.9	13.2	7.9
Grain crisps	6 crisps	90	4.3	.3	24
Carrot juice	8 ounces	53	4.8	.7	29
Cauliflower loaf	1½ cups	209	17.2	11.7	36.6
Hippocrates salad	1 serving	80	5.6	1.2	18
Avocado-tomato dressing	½ cup	200	3.2	16.6	11
Basic bread	2 slices	150	6.1	5	34
Rejuvelac with honey	8 ounces 2 tablespoons	221	1.2	trace	12.3
TOTALS		2033	78.9	53.3	312.9

* (see p. 174)

Calcium	Phosphorus	Iron	Sodium	Potassium	Vitamin A	Vitamin B_1 (thiamine)	Vitamin B_2 (riboflavin)	Niacin	Vitamin C (ascorbic acid)
Milligrams					**I.U.**	**Milligrams**			
29.1	190	2.4	680	120	0	.1	trace	.1	14
5	5.5	.4	.5	220	115	.03	.04	.4	6
73	139	1.5	7	101	0	.07	.15	1.1	2.1
25	40	1.5	11	300	7	.04	.05	.2	.5
536.5	**1370.5**	**23.1**	**140.5**	**3970**	**6556**	**1.36**	**.82**	**4.2**	**65**
160.1	101	3.4	60.2	1006	9056.2	.32	.33	1.9	82.1
84.7	103	1.2	.8	184	trace	.1	.23	1.9	3
48	142	1.6	1.5	145	trace	.18	.06	1.6	trace
162	141	2.2	229	1400	19460	.22	.21	5.4	53
138	215	5.2	10.6	878	40	.32	.51	4.6	9
160.1	101	3.4	60.2	1006	9056.2	.32	.33	1.9	82.1
23	69	1.1	7	848	1190	.17	.24	2.3	37
62	191	2.1	2.6	239	trace	.37	.12	2.1	trace
29	7.9	.5	10	64	trace	trace	.09	.7	trace
1535.5	**2815.9**	**49.5**	**1220.9**	**10481**	**45480.4**	**3.60**	**3.17**	**28.3**	**353.8**

SUMMARY—

TYPICAL HIPPOCRATES DIET MENU TOTALS COMPARED TO THE 1980 RDAs

Category	Group	Calories (actual)‡	Protein	Fat	Carbohydrate
Measurement Units			**Grams**		
Hippocrates Diet Totals*	all	2033	78.9	53.3	312.9
U.S. RDAs† Males	ages 23-50	2381	56	—	—
U.S. RDAs† Females	ages 23-50	1565	44	—	—

Note: a dash means that there is no official RDA for that nutrient.

Sources:
* Estimated nutritional content of the Hippocrates Diet is based on *USDA Composition of Foods Handbook No. 8.*

† The figures used were established by the U.S. Food and Drug Administration in 1980.

‡ Data on American calorie intake is from *USDA Nationwide Food Comparison Survey, 1977-78*, issued by the United States Department of Agriculture.

Calcium	Phosphorus	Iron	Sodium	Potassium	Vitamin A	Vitamin B_1 (thiamine)	Vitamin B_2 (riboflavin)	Niacin	Vitamin C (ascorbic acid)
Milligrams					**I.U.**		**Milligrams**		
1535.5	2815.9	49.5	1220.9	10481	45480.4	3.60	3.17	28.3	353.8
800	800	10	—	—	5000	1.4	1.6	18	60
800	800	10	—	—	5000	1.0	1.2	13	60

COMPOSITION OF FOODS, 100 GRAMS, EDIBLE PORTIONS, 3½ OZ.

Foods	Protein	Fat	Carbohydrate	Calcium	Phosphorus
Measurement Units	Grams	Grams	Grams	Mg	Mg
Almonds	18.6	54.2	19.5	234	504
Apples	.2	.6	14.5	7	10
Apricots	1.0	.2	12.8	17	23
Asparagus	2.5	.2	5.0	22	62
Avocados	2.1	16.4	6.3	10	42
Bananas	1.1	.2	22.2	8	26
Barley	8.2	1.0	78.8	16	189
Beans (Mung)	24.2	1.3	60.3	118	340
Beans (Green)	1.9	.2	7.1	56	44
Beans (Mung sprouts)	3.8	.2	6.6	19	64
Beet (Red)	1.6	.1	9.9	16	33
Beet (Greens)	2.2	.3	4.6	119	40
Blackberries	1.2	.9	12.9	32	19
Blueberries	.7	.5	15.3	15	13
Cabbage	1.3	.2	5.4	49	29
Carrots	1.1	.2	9.7	37	36
Cauliflower	2.7	.2	5.2	25	56
Celery	.9	.1	3.9	39	28
Chard (Swiss)	2.4	.3	4.6	88	39
Cherries (Sweet)	1.3	.3	17.4	22	19
Chives	1.8	.3	5.8	69	44
Collards	4.8	.8	7.5	250	82
Corn (Sweet)	3.5	1.0	22.1	3	111

Iron	Sodium	Potassium	Vitamin A	Vitamin B_1 (thiamine)	Vitamin B_2 (riboflavin)	Niacin	Vitamin C (ascorbic acid)
Mg	Mg	Mg	Mg	I.U.	Mg	Mg	Mg
4.7	4	773	0	.24	.92	3.5	trace
.3	1	110	90	.03	.02	.1	4
.5	1	281	2700	.03	.04	.6	10
1.0	2	278	900	.18	.20	1.5	33
.6	4	604	290	.11	.20	1.6	14
.7	1	370	190	.05	.06	.7	10
2.0	3	160	0	.12	.05	3.1	0
7.7	6	1028	80	.38	.21	2.6	—
.8	7	243	600	.08	.11	.5	19
1.3	5	223	20	.13	.13	.8	19
.7	60	335	20	.03	.05	.4	10
3.3	130	570	6100	.10	.22	.4	30
.9	1	170	200	.03	.04	.4	21
1.0	1	81	100	.03	.06	.5	14
.4	20	233	130	.05	.05	.3	47
.7	47	341	11000	.06	.05	.6	8
1.1	13	295	60	.11	.10	.7	78
.3	126	341	240	.03	.03	.3	9
3.2	147	550	6500	.06	.17	.5	32
.4	2	191	110	.05	.06	.4	10
1.7	—	250	5800	.08	.13	.5	56
1.5	—	450	9300	.16	.31	1.7	152
.7	trace	280	400	.15	.12	1.7	12

COMPOSITION OF FOODS, continued

Foods	Protein	Fat	Carbohydrate	Calcium	Phosphorus
Measurement Units	Grams	Grams	Grams	Mg	Mg
Cow peas	9.0	.8	21.8	27	172
Dulse	—	3.2	—	296	267
Endive	1.7	.1	4.1	81	54
Figs	1.2	.3	20.3	35	22
Garlic	6.2	.2	30.8	29	202
Gooseberries	.8	.2	9.7	18	15
Grapefruit	.5	.1	10.6	16	16
Grapes	1.3	.1	15.7	16	12
Guavas	.8	.6	15.0	23	42
Kale	6.0	.8	9.0	249	93
Kelp	—	1.1	—	1093	240
Kumquats	.9	.1	17.1	63	23
Leeks	2.2	.3	11.2	52	50
Lemons	1.1	.3	8.2	26	16
Lentils	24.7	1.1	60.1	79	377
Lettuce	1.2	.2	2.5	35	26
Mushrooms	2.7	.3	4.4	6	116
Muskmelons	.7	.1	7.5	14	16
Mustard greens	3.0	.5	5.6	183	50
Nectarines	.6	trace	17.1	4	24
Onions (Dry)	1.5	.1	8.7	27	36
Onions (Green)	1.5	.2	8.2	51	39
Oranges	1.0	.2	12.2	41	20

Iron	Sodium	Potassium	Vitamin A	Vitamin B_1 (thiamine)	Vitamin B_2 (riboflavin)	Niacin	Vitamin C (ascorbic acid)
Mg	Mg	Mg	Mg	I.U.	Mg	Mg	Mg
2.3	2	541	370	.43	.13	1.6	29
—	2085	8060	—	—	—	—	—
1.7	14	294	3300	.07	.14	.5	10
.6	2	194	80	.06	.05	.4	2
1.5	19	529	trace	.25	.08	.5	15
.5	1	155	290	—	—	—	33
.4	1	135	80	.04	.02	.2	38
.4	3	158	100	.05	.03	.3	4
.9	4	289	280	.05	.05	1.2	242
2.7	75	378	10000	.16	.26	2.1	186
—	3007	5273	—	—	—	—	—
.4	7	236	600	.08	.10	—	36
1.1	5	347	40	.11	.06	.5	17
.6	2	138	20	.04	.02	.1	53
6.8	30	790	60	.37	.22	2.0	—
2.0	9	264	970	.06	.06	.3	8
.8	15	414	trace	.10	.46	4.2	3
.4	12	251	3400	.04	.03	.6	33
3.0	32	377	7000	.11	.22	.8	97
.5	6	294	1650	—	—	—	13
.5	10	157	40	.03	.04	.2	10
1.0	5	231	2000	.05	.05	.4	32
.4	1	200	200	.10	.04	.4	50

COMPOSITION OF FOODS, continued

Foods	Protein	Fat	Carbohydrate	Calcium	Phosphorus
Measurement Units	Grams	Grams	Grams	Mg	Mg
Papayas	.6	.1	10.0	20	16
Parsley	3.6	.6	8.5	203	63
Parsnips	1.7	.5	17.5	50	77
Peaches	.6	.1	9.7	9	19
Peanuts (Raw)	26.0	47.5	18.6	69	401
Pears	.7	.4	15.3	8	11
Peas (Edible Pod)	3.4	.2	12.0	62	90
Peas (Green)	6.3	.4	14.4	26	116
Pecans	9.2	71.2	14.6	73	289
Peppers (Hot red)	3.7	2.3	18.1	29	78
Peppers (Sweet green)	1.2	.2	4.8	9	22
Persimmons	.7	.4	19.7	6	26
Pineapple	.4	.2	13.7	17	8
Plums	.5	trace	17.8	18	17
Pomegranate	.5	.3	16.4	3	8
Rye	12.1	1.7	73.4	38	376
Sesame Seeds	18.6	49.1	21.6	1160	616
Soybeans	10.9	5.1	13.2	67	225
Spinach	3.2	.3	4.3	93	51
Squash	1.1	.1	4.2	28	29
Strawberries	.7	.5	8.4	21	21
Sunflower Seeds	24.0	47.3	19.9	120	837
Tangerines	.8	.2	11.6	40	18

Iron	Sodium	Potassium	Vitamin A	Vitamin B_1 (thiamine)	Vitamin B_2 (riboflavin)	Niacin	Vitamin C (ascorbic acid)
Mg	Mg	Mg	Mg	I.U.	Mg	Mg	Mg
.3	3	234	1750	.04	.04	.3	56
6.2	45	727	8500	.12	.26	1.2	172
.7	12	541	30	.08	.09	.2	16
.5	1	202	1330	.02	.05	1.0	7
2.1	5	674	—	1.14	.13	17.2	0
.3	2	130	20	.02	.04	.1	4
.7	—	170	680	.28	.12	—	21
1.9	2	316	640	.35	.14	2.9	27
2.4	trace	603	130	.86	.13	.9	2
1.2	—	—	21600	.22	.36	4.4	369
.7	13	213	420	.08	.08	.5	128
.3	6	174	2700	.03	.02	.1	11
.5	1	146	70	.09	.03	.2	17
.5	2	299	300	.08	.03	.5	—
.3	3	259	trace	.03	.03	.3	4
3.7	1	467	0	.43	.22	1.6	0
10.5	60	725	30	.98	.24	5.4	0
2.8	—	—	690	.44	.16	1.4	29
3.1	71	470	8100	.10	.20	.6	51
.4	1	202	410	.05	.09	1.0	22
1.0	1	164	60	.03	.07	.6	59
7.1	30	920	50	1.96	.23	5.4	—
.4	2	126	420	.06	.02	.1	31

COMPOSITION OF FOODS, continued

Foods	Protein	Fat	Carbohydrate	Calcium	Phosphorus
Measurement Units	**Grams**	**Grams**	**Grams**	**Mg**	**Mg**
Tomatoes	1.1	.2	4.7	13	27
Turnips	1.0	.2	6.6	39	30
Turnip (Greens)	3.0	.3	5.0	246	58
Vinegar (Apple Cider)	trace	0	5.9	6	9
Walnuts (English)	14.8	64.0	15.8	99	380
Watercress	2.2	.3	3.0	151	54
Watermelon	.5	.2	6.4	7	10
Wheat (Hard red winter)	12.3	1.8	71.7	46	354
Wheat (Soft spring white)	9.4	2.0	75.4	36	394

Source: *Composition of Foods Handbook No. 8, United States Department of Agriculture.*

Iron	Sodium	Potassium	Vitamin A	Vitamin B_1 (thiamine)	Vitamin B_2 (riboflavin)	Niacin	Vitamin C (ascorbic acid)
Mg	Mg	Mg	Mg	I.U.	Mg	Mg	Mg
.5	3	244	900	.06	.04	.7	23
.5	49	268	trace	.04	.07	.6	36
1.8	—	—	7600	.21	.39	.8	139
.6	1	100	—	—	—	—	—
3.1	2	450	30	.33	.13	.9	2
1.7	52	282	4900	.08	.16	.9	79
.5	1	100	590	.03	.03	.2	7
3.4	3	370	0	.52	.12	4.3	0
3.0	3	390	0	.53	.12	5.3	0

Appendix B

HIPPOCRATES DIET SUPPLIES AND INFORMATION

The Hippocrates Health Institute is a pioneer in the field of self-help care. Since 1963, our program has been helping thousands of people like yourself take responsibility for being healthy and happy—and for staying that way.

Whatever the cause, we can help you with your present problem—before it leads to more serious complications. Our goal is to assist you in isolating, understanding and removing the weights that may be dragging you down, thus helping to improve your condition. We help you:

- Look and feel better
- Get the most from, and increase, your present energy and alertness levels
- Rebuild, regenerate, recharge, and rejuvenate your body and mind
- Experience the sensation of self-sufficiency
- Complement your current health/medical program

We feel that, inside all of us, a "natural healer" awaits the call. Our health professionals help awaken your inner resources and strengthen them by teaching you new health-inducing styles of eating, thinking and living—to help you change your lifestyle for a lifetime.

The Hippocrates approach emphasizes the need to nurture and transform the whole you—body, mind, emotions, and spirit. Because true health and vitality are merely reflections of the harmony and balance between your physical, mental and spiritual aspects.

Helping you to better health is what the Hippocrates program and faculty are all about. For more information about the Hippocrates program, other books in the Hippocrates Health Series, a list of live food equipment, supplies, and health aids available, call or write to:

Ann Wigmore Institute
P.O. Box 429
Rincon, PR 00677
(787) 868-6307 phone
(787) 868-2430 fax

Ann Wigmore Foundation
P.O. Box 399
San Fidel, NM 87049
(505) 552-0595

Index